Bridget Simon
CERTIFIED JUICE THERAPIST

MAMA'S HEALTHY KITCHEN

Life Restoration Program

Mama's Healthy Kitchen
Copyright © 2025 by Bridget Simon

All rights reserved. No part of this publication may be reproduced, distributed, or transmitted in any form or by any means, including photocopying, recording, or other electronic or mechanical methods, without the prior written permission of the copyright holder, except in the case of brief quotations embodied in critical reviews and certain other noncommercial uses permitted by copyright law. For permission requests, write to the publisher, addressed "Attention: Permissions Coordinator," at the address below.

Soft Cover – 978-1-64318-140-0

Imperium Publishing
1097 N. 400th Rd
Baldwin City, KS, 66006

www.imperiumpublishing.com

A SPECIAL THANKS

James, Holly, and their family are outstanding individuals who have made a significant positive impact on my life. Their support has been multifaceted, ranging from chiropractic care at Thrive Family Chiropractor to the opening of IV Nutrition-St. Joseph, MO. Their generosity and dedication to helping others are inspiring qualities that they consistently exhibit.

What they have to say:

"Thank you for the food!! All delicious, as usual."
"This Spinach Chicken Spaghetti is GREAT!!"
"As always your food is delicious and nourishing."
—James and Holly Schoonover

I advise to use as much organic as possible on all recipes! Look for USDA Certified labs. *Violife* products are a good brand for dairy and gluten-free butter, sour cream, cream cheese, cheeses and other products. But any products you can find that are dairy-free and gluten-free will work.

CONTENTS

My Story 9

Breakfast Meals & Smoothies 11
    Vanilla Chia Seed Pudding (2 Servings) 12
    Banana and Cream "N" Oatmeal 13
    Chicken Breakfast Hash 14
    Turkey Breakfast Sausages 15
    Veggie Omelet 16
    Vegetable Egg Muffin 17
    Who said you can't have Cake for breakfast? 18

Smoothies 21
    Smoothie #1: Green Lymphatic Detox 22
    Smoothie #2: Avocado Berry Blast 23
    Smoothie #3: Minty Green Delight 24
    Smoothie #4: Berry Butter 25
    Smoothie #5: Kiwi Banana Blast 26
    Smoothie #6: Bubble Gum Blast 27
    Smoothie #7: Belly Burner 28

Bonus Drinks For Certain Health Issues 29
    Homemade Hydrating Electrolyte Drink 30
    Inflammation Reducer 31
    Lung Support / Health 32
    Heart Health Drink 33

Salads 35
    Crunchy Detox Salad 36
    Mediterranean Salad 38
    Basil Mint Fruit Salad 40

Soups Recipes 41
    Enchilada Soup 42
    Chicken Pot Pie Soup 44
    Pasta Fagioli Soup 46
    Easy Bison Soup 47
    Creamy Chicken Soup 48
    Chicken Ginger Soup 50
    Taco Soup 52
    Notes: 54

Entrees 57
    Smothered Spinach Chicken 58
    Chicken with Garlic Parmesan Rice 59
    Veggie Sweet N' Sour Chicken 61
    Homemade Chicken Helper Meal 62
    Homemade Bison Helper Meal 64
    Crispy Mushroom Toast with Ricotta 66
    Italian Chicken Zucchini Pizza 68
    Sweet & Smoky Jalapeño Stuff Chicken 69
    Chicken Bacon Ranch Roll-Ups 71
    Stuffed Jalapeño Turkey Breast 72

Bison Meatloaf Dish	73
Teriyaki Chicken Lettuce Wraps	74
Gobbler Poppers	76
Homemade Sloppy Joe	78
Garlic Honey Salmon with Asparagus	79
Garlic Butter Chicken Bites with Lemon Asparagus	81
Bacon Guacamole Grilled Cheese Sandwich	83
Green Smothered Chicken	84
Garlic Parmesan Chicken Skewers	85
Veggie Chicken or Turkey Dish	86
Stuffed Poblano Peppers	87
Chicken and Avocado Enchiladas in Creamy Avocado Sauce	89
Spinach Garlic Meatballs Stuffed With Mozzarella	91
Chicken or Turkey Breast Stuffin'	93
Creamy Garlic Parmesan Mushrooms	94
Teriyaki Chicken Pan	95
Slow Cooker BBQ Honey Garlic Chicken	97
Cheesy Garlic Zucchini Steaks	99
Pineapple Chicken and Rice	101
Garlic Mushrooms Cauliflower Skillet	103
Crispy Broccoli Cheese Bites	105
Garlic Chicken Fried Rice	106
Grilled Salmon Skewers with Creamy Dill Yogurt Sauce	108
Spinach Ricotta Stuffed Chicken Breasts	110
Zucchini Pizza Bites	111
Mediterranean Chicken Zucchini Bake	112
Honey Pineapple Jalapeño Salmon	114
Creamy Spinach Tomato Spaghetti	116
Chicken Mushroom and Spinach Lasagna	118
Mushroom Ravioli with Spinach	120
Marinade Recipes for Chicken	121

Desserts & Snacks................................123
    Fruit Protein Balls 124
    Your Mango Cheesecake Delight 125
    Cherry Cheesecake Fluff........................126
    Fruit Bliss Cheesecake 128
    Brownie Bombs 130
    Caramel Cheesecake Bars........................132
    White Chocolate Strawberry Cheesecake Bites...........134

MY STORY

"*I'm just so exhausted,* all I wanna do is sleep."

"I wish I knew what was going on with my belly. It hurts like somebody's stabbed me. It's so swollen…"

"Why can't my bowels make up their minds? I'm either going nonstop or nothing happens for days no matter what I take. I don't want to eat 'cause I don't know what's gonna happen."

"I can't breathe. My head is so congested, but nothing comes out."

"My chest can stop feeling like this anytime. My lung(s) are on fire and it hurts to breathe."

Every time I thought I had found a pattern, my body proved me wrong. I was done living in this unpredictable cycle. It was time to surrender to the fact that my body was changing without my permission. My journey of healing began. Traditional medicine, holistic practitioners, God, anything that could offer me some type of relief was welcome. Nutrition has been a cornerstone to change. Through countless hours of research, networking, and trial & error, I have been able to put together this book of successful recipes that have complimented my healing and nourished my soul in the process. The journey is not over. As I move forward, I invite you to join in my success, and I offer you an easy-to-implement way to bring healing to your own home.

BREAKFAST MEALS & SMOOTHIES

I prefer a simple approach! With hectic and crazy mornings, starting the day with a smoothie, chia pudding, or a veggie egg muffin is the perfect, effortless way to begin. Reserve your weekends for more substantial meals. When the children are home, I enjoy preparing a variety, as I am not eating alone or rushing to ensure everyone has everything needed for the day. This provides the perfect boost for a healthy start, preparing you to face the day ahead, and giving you those omega-3s first thing any day.

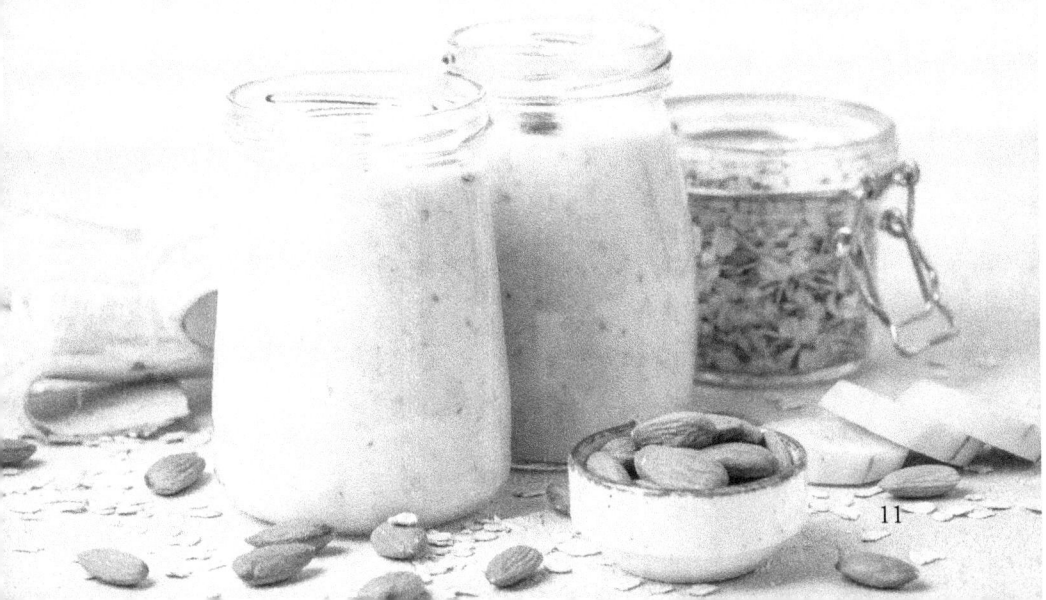

VANILLA CHIA SEED PUDDING (2 SERVINGS)

Ingredients:

- 2 cups of any of these milks — Coconut, Flaxseed, or Almond (I use vanilla almond milk.)
- 2 Tbsp. grade A or B maple syrup
- 1/2 tsp. pure vanilla extract (optional)
- 1/2 cup chia seeds or
- 1/4 cup chia seeds and 1/4 cup flaxseeds

Directions:

Mix ingredients together. Cover and refrigerate for at least 3 hours or overnight. Serve with your choice of fruit (bananas, blueberries, raspberries, plums, peaches, kiwi, etc.).

Add yogurt if you choose. Preferably coconut yogurt.

BANANA AND CREAM "N" OATMEAL

Ingredients:

- 2 ripe bananas
- 4 Tbsp. coconut or almond butter or *Violife* butter
- 2 pinches of sea salt
- 1/2 tsp. of cinnamon, nutmeg or pumpkin spice

Directions:

Mash banana. Add the sea salt and cinnamon, nutmeg, or pumpkin spice. Warm the butter in a sauce pan over low heat. When it's runny and warm, remove from heat and scoop it into the banana mixture.

CHICKEN BREAKFAST HASH

Ingredients:

- 1 lb. organic chicken, shredded
- Olive oil spray
- 3 garlic cloves, minced
- 1/2 of a green, red, yellow, orange pepper (optional, can add all)
- 1/4 cup cheese of choice (*Violife* cheddar preferred)
- 1/2 Shallot onion, minced
- 6 organic eggs
- 1 tsp. thyme
- 1 tsp. rosemary
- Sea salt or Mediterranean salt, and black pepper to taste.

Directions:

Cook chicken in oven for 30 minutes and shred once cooled (can always cook beforehand). Spray olive oil in a spread pan (skillet), and cook garlic, peppers, onion, thyme and rosemary until slightly tender. Whisk eggs in a bowl. Add chicken and eggs to skillet that has your herbs, garlic, peppers and onion. Let cook until eggs are done.

TURKEY BREAKFAST SAUSAGES

Ingredients:

- 1 lb. ground turkey
- 2 tsp. fresh sage (or 1 tsp. dried)
- 1 tsp. fresh rosemary (or 1/2 tsp. dried)
- 1 tsp. fresh thyme (or 1/2 tsp. dried)
- 1/2 tsp. garlic powder
- 1/2 tsp. cinnamon or nutmeg
- 1 tsp. sea salt or Celtic salt
- 2 Tbsp. of coconut oil or avocado oil

Directions:

Combine all ingredients except the oil and refrigerate for 30 mins. Add the oil and shape into patties. Cook in a lightly oiled skillet on medium heat or bake at 400F for 25 minutes.

VEGGIE OMELET

Ingredients:

- 1-2 tsp. avocado oil
- 1 cup broccoli, carrots, or cauliflower
- 1 cup mushrooms, chopped
- 1/2 shallot onion (or your choice), chopped
- 8 eggs (preferably organic)
- Sea salt and black pepper to taste

Directions:

Add oil to pan. Add chopped broccoli, carrots or cauliflower, onion, and mushrooms to cook on medium heat for 8-10 mins. Whisk eggs in a bowl, then put in skillet with veggies. Cook until done. Feel free to top with cheese of your choice or avocado slices, and fold over for omelet.

VEGETABLE EGG MUFFIN

Ingredients:

- 8 whole eggs
- 1/2 cup yellow onion, minced
- 1/2 cup mushrooms, minced
- 1 cup spinach, chopped
- 1 Tbsp. coconut or avocado oil
- 1-2 garlic cloves, minced
- 2 Tbsp. fresh chives, minced (or can use 1 Tbsp. dried)
- 1 Tbsp. Parsley (or can use 1/2 Tbsp. dried)
- Sea salt and black pepper to taste

Directions:

Preheat oven to 350°. Over medium heat in skillet, melt oil and cook onion and garlic for 3-4 minutes. Add other veggies and herbs, and cook until soft.

Grease muffin pan, spoon the cooked veggies in each muffin tin. Whisk eggs in bowl with seasonings, then add to top of veggies and bake 15-18 minutes.

WHO SAID YOU CAN'T HAVE CAKE FOR BREAKFAST?

Ingredients:

- 1 1/4 cups sweet potato, cubed
- 1 1/4 cups apple, cored & cubed
- 1 cup milk (coconut or almond)
- 2 large eggs
- 1/4 cup maple syrup or honey
- 1 tsp. pure vanilla extract
- 1/2 tsp. baking powder
- 1/2 tsp. baking soda
- 1/4 tsp. salt
- 2 1/2 cups rolled oats or quick oats
- 2 Tbsp. nuts for garnish (cashews recommended)
- 2 Tbsp. coconut flakes or almond flakes for garnish (optional)
- Cooking spray for greasing

Directions:

Preheat oven to 375°, and spray a pie baking dish with cooking spray. Set aside.

In a high-speed blender, add sweet potato, apple, milk, eggs, maple syrup, vanilla, baking powder, baking soda, salt, and oats. Blend until apples and sweet potato are finely ground and everything is well combined, about 30 seconds. Pour the batter into the prepared baking dish. Tap to level, and sprinkle with nuts and flakes. Bake for 40 minutes or until a toothpick inserted in the center comes out clean. Remove from the oven, and let cool for 20 minutes.

Cut into 8 slices. Serve warm on its own or with a dollop of Greek yogurt and a drizzle of honey or maple syrup.

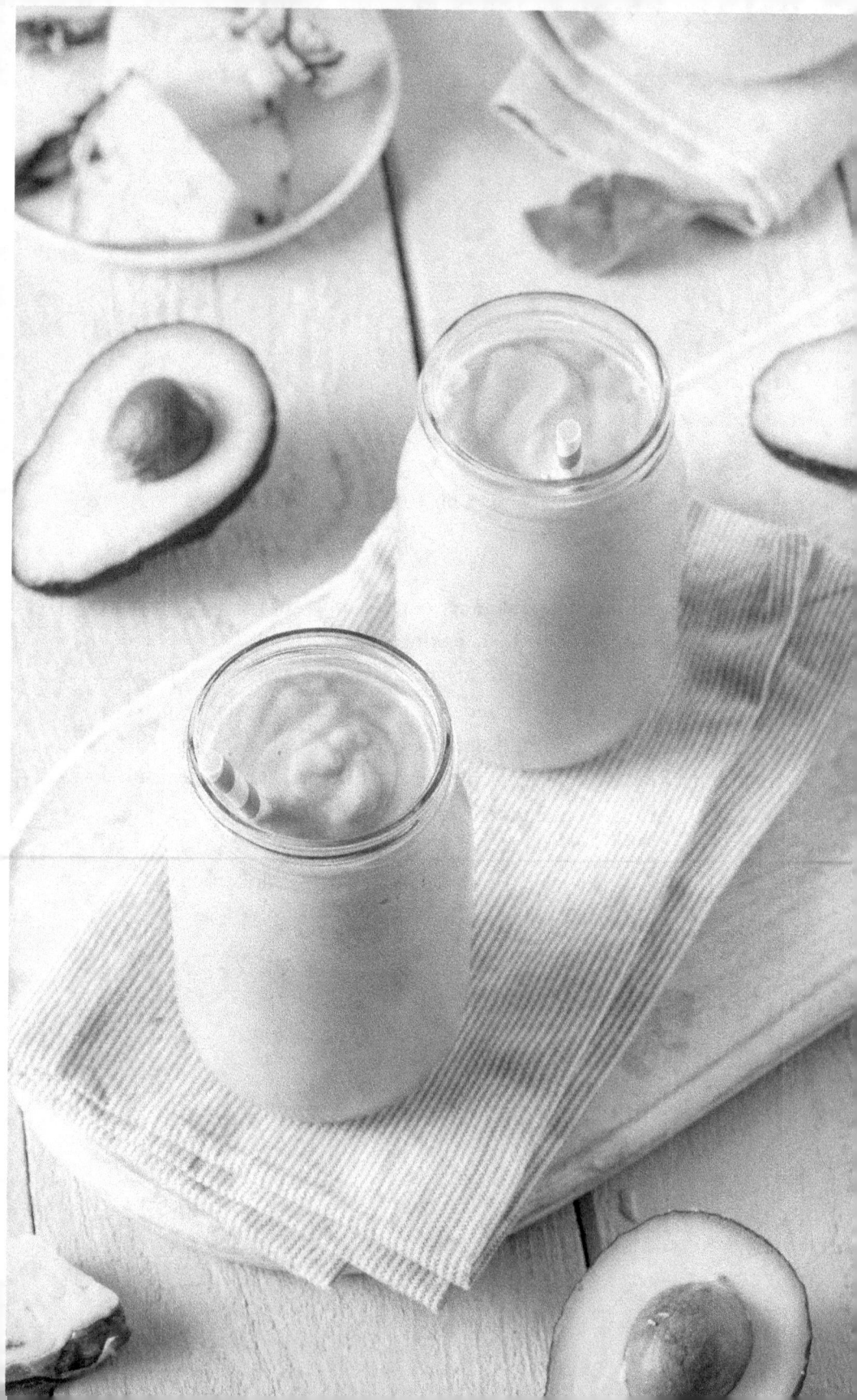

SMOOTHIES

My mornings had to change, and I had to start eating something rather than nothing. Smoothies were the best option for me that helped keep my blood sugars where they needed to be and my body feeling supported with the right nutrition.

SMOOTHIE #1: GREEN LYMPHATIC DETOX

Ingredients:

- 1 green apple
- 1/2 cucumber, peeled
- Juice of 1/2 lemon
- Juice of 1/2 lime
- 1 Tbsp. fresh ginger, chopped
- 1 cup kale
- 1 cup of coconut or almond milk
- 1 Tbsp. *Moringa Powder*
- 1 scoop protein powder (*Organic Garden of Life* recommended)

Blend until well mixed together.

SMOOTHIE #2: AVOCADO BERRY BLAST

Ingredients:

- 1/2 avocado
- 1 cup frozen berries (mixture of choice)
- 1 cup coconut or almond milk (flavored optional)
- 2 cups leafy greens
- 1 Tbsp. *Moringa Powder*
- 1 Tbsp. of *Mega Mushroom Powder*
- 1 scoop protein powder (*Organic Garden of Life* recommended)

Blend until well mixed together.

SMOOTHIE #3: MINTY GREEN DELIGHT

Ingredients:

- 1 frozen banana
- 1 cup fresh spinach
- 1/4 avocado
- 1 cup coconut or almond milk
- 1 tsp. peppermint extract or a small handful of mint leafs
- 1 tsp. raw local honey or maple syrup
- 1 Tbsp. *Moringa Powder*
- 1 scoop protein powder (*Organic Garden of Life* recommended)
- Handful of ice cubes

Blend until well mixed together.

SMOOTHIE #4: BERRY BUTTER

Ingredients:

- 1 cup mixed berries
- 2 Tbsp. nut butter (or seed butter)
- 1-2 cups coconut or almond milk (flavored optional)
- 1 cup leafy greens
- 1 Tbsp. *Mega Mushroom Powder*
- 1 scoop protein powder (*Organic Garden of Life* recommended)

Blend until well mixed together.

SMOOTHIE #5: KIWI BANANA BLAST

Ingredients:

- 1/2 cup spinach
- 1/4 cup kiwi or 1 full kiwi
- 1/2 banana
- 1 Tbsp. chia seeds
- 1 Tbsp. of total omega - *Barlean's* brand
- 1 cup of *GoodBelly Probiotics Juice**
- 1 scoop protein powder (*Organic Garden of Life* recommended)*

Blend until well mixed together.

*Found at Sprout's, Natural Grocers, Trader Joe's or any Whole Health store.

SMOOTHIE #6: BUBBLE GUM BLAST

Ingredients:

- 1/2 cup spinach
- 1/2 cup kale
- 1/4 cup Blueberries
- 1/2 a banana
- 1 Tbsp. chia seeds
- 1 Tbsp. of total omega - *Barlean's* brand
- 1 cup of *GoodBelly Probiotics Juice**
- 1 scoop protein powder (*Organic Garden of Life* recommended)*

Blend until well mixed together.

*Found at Sprout's, Natural Grocers, or Trader Joe's.

SMOOTHIE #7: BELLY BURNER

Ingredients:

- 1/2 cup spinach
- 1/3 cup kale
- 1/2 a banana
- 1/2 cup mixed berries
- 1 Tbsp. chia seeds
- 1 Tbsp. hemp seeds
- 1 Tbsp. of total omega
- 1 cup of *GoodBelly Probiotics Juice**
- 1 scoop protein powder (*Organic Garden of Life* recommended)*

Blend until well mixed together.

Mixed with high fiber, great omega's and probiotics, this will have your body craving more while leaving you full for longer. Great breakfast or lunch.

*Found at Sprout's, Natural Grocers, or Trader Joe's.

BONUS DRINKS FOR CERTAIN HEALTH ISSUES

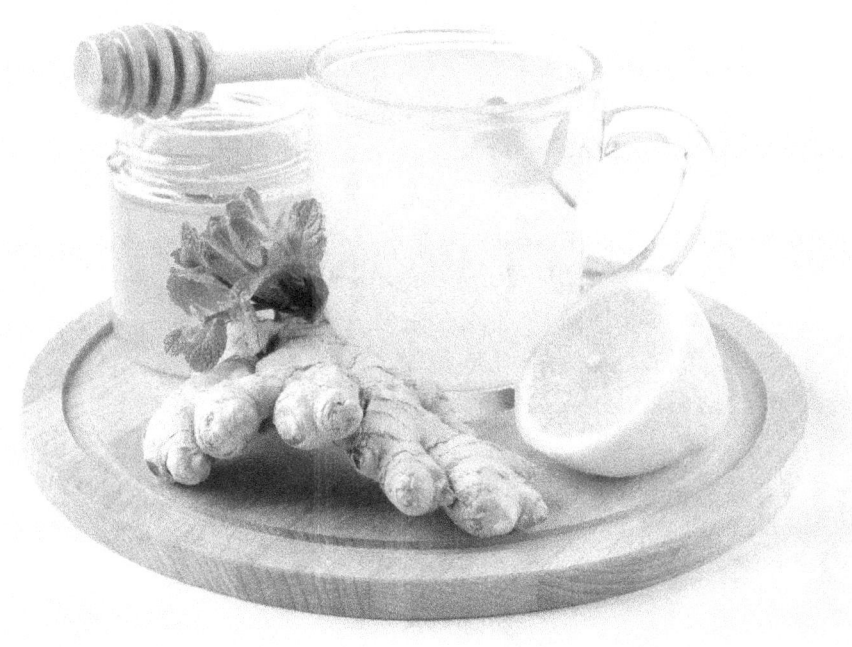

HOMEMADE HYDRATING ELECTROLYTE DRINK

Ingredients:

- 16 oz. pure water
- 4 oz. freshly squeezed lemon or lime juice
- 1/8 tsp. *Celtic Salt*
- Add 1/4 Tbsp. raw honey or 2 Tbsp. of maple syrup to taste if desired.

Directions:

Combine ingredients and enjoy at least once daily.

This is great for many reasons and has tons of benefits. I made it up for a friend when she was super ill and her direct message to me when I checked on her later was "I don't know what's in that drink, but my head isn't pounding like it was, and I don't think I'd be feeling as good as what I do if you hadn't done this for me."

INFLAMMATION REDUCER

Ingredients:

- 1 Turmeric, peeled and sliced
- 1/4 ginger root, peeled and sliced
- 1 lemon, squeezed
- 1 grapefruit, squeezed
- 1/3 cup raw honey
- 1/2 bottle *Icelandic* water
- 1 Tbsp. *Chaga* mushroom power

Directions:

Combine all ingredients in a pot on the stove on medium heat and let simmer for 15 minutes. Then drain or blend once cooled and enjoy.

One of my favorites. Bye bye inflammation!

LUNG SUPPORT / HEALTH

Ingredients:

- 1 Turmeric, peeled and sliced
- 1/4 ginger root, peeled and sliced
- 1 lemon squeezed
- 1 lime squeezed
- 1/3 cup raw honey
- 1/2 bottle *Icelandic* water or similar
- 1 Tbsp. *Chaga* mushroom powder
- 1 Tbsp. *Tiger Milk* mushroom powder
- 1 Tbsp. mullein leaf

Directions:

Combine all ingredients in a pot on the stove on medium heat and let simmer for 15 minutes. Then drain or blend once cooled and enjoy.

HEART HEALTH DRINK

Ingredients:

- 1/3 cup frozen organic spinach
- 1/3 cup frozen organic avocado
- 1/3 cup frozen organic green apple
- 1/3 cup frozen organic papaya
- 1/3 cup frozen organic pomegranate
- 1 Tbsp. beet powder or 3/4 cup organic beet juice (*Beetology* is recommended)
- 1/2 tsp. maple syrup if desired

Directions:

If you don't use beet juice, add *Icelandic* water and blend to smoothie or liquid style of choice, and enjoy.

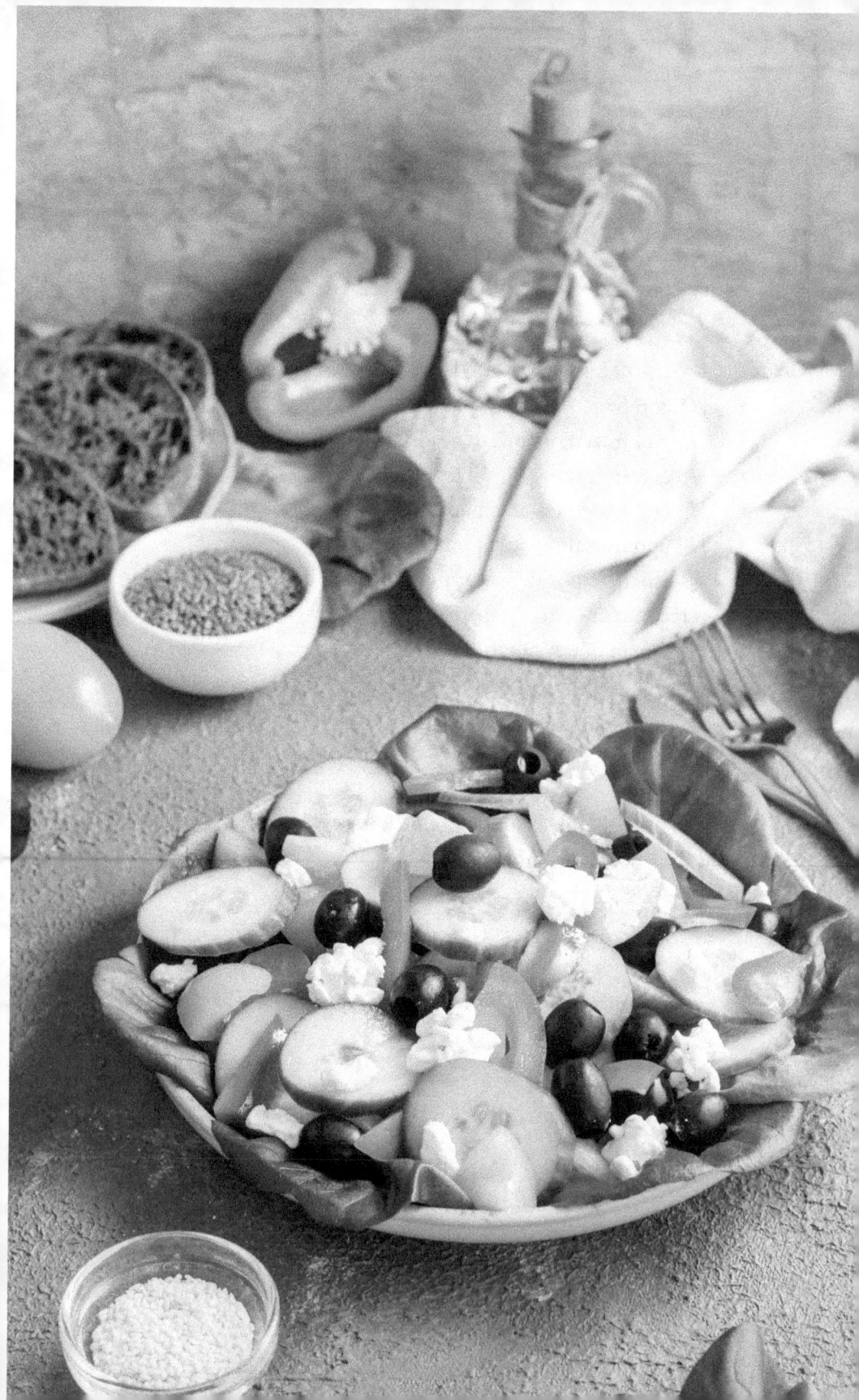

SALADS

Maintaining physical balance at an optimal level can be a considerable challenge without the consumption of nutritious foods. In my case, the management of multiple health concerns required a comprehensive overhaul of my lifestyle—incorporating healthy habits and nutritious meals. Given my heightened risk for lung diseases, heart disease, and diabetes, this transformation was vital. To facilitate this process, my goal was to create three new, healthy recipes daily over the course of several months. The ultimate goal was to compile a guide to support others at risk for lung diseases, heart disease, diabetes, and other health issues, with all meals being dairy-free, gluten-free and composed of non- processed, organic foods.

CRUNCHY DETOX SALAD

Ingredients:

- 2 cups cauliflower, chopped
- 2 cups broccoli, chopped
- 1 cup red cabbage, chopped
- 1 cup carrots, chopped
- 1-1/2 cups fresh parsley, chopped
- 2 celery stalks, chopped
- 1/2 cup almonds, chopped
- 1/2 cup sunflower seeds
- 1/3 cup organic raisins

Directions:

Either chop the ingredients using a good sharp knife, or toss them individually in a food processor and pulse a few times so they are finely chopped. Add all of the salad ingredients to a large bowl and toss with the vinaigrette.

Vinaigrette:

- 3 Tbsps. olive oil
- 1/2 cup lemon juice
- 1 Tbsp. fresh ginger, peeled and grated
- 2 Tbsps. clover honey
- 1/2 tsp. sea salt

Place the ingredients for the vinaigrette in a mason jar and seal the lid. Shake well. You can also place the ingredients in a small bowl and whisk to blend. Best if refrigerated for up to an hour before use.

MEDITERRANEAN SALAD

Ingredients:

- 1/2 cup Romaine lettuce
- 1/2 cup spinach leafs
- 1/4 cup kale
- 1/4 cup salad tomatoes (halves)
- 1/4 cup baby cucumbers (sliced thin)
- 1/4 cup red onions (sliced thin)
- 1/4 cup Kalamata olives (halves)
- 1/4 cup chickpeas
- 1/4 cup bell peppers (sliced thin)
- 1/4 cup feta cheese crumbled
- 1/3 cup freshly chopped parsley

Directions:

Combine all ingredients in a salad bowl or tray. Top with a lemon vinaigrette dressing.

Vinaigrette:

- 1/4 cup fresh lemon juice
- 1 tsp. garlic clove
- 1 tsp. Dijon mustard
- 1/3 cup extra virgin olive oil
- 1/2 tsp. honey or maple syrup
- 1/3 tsp. dried oregano
- Sea salt and black pepper to taste

BASIL MINT FRUIT SALAD

Ingredients:

- 1/2 a head of lettuce (chopped)
- 1/2 fresh mint - found in most grocery stores
- 1/2 fresh basil - found in most grocery stores
- 1 cup watermelon (small cubes)
- 1 cup strawberries (small cubes)
- 1 banana (thinly sliced)
- 2 mandarin oranges or 1/2 can (small cubes)
- 1 cup green or purple grapes (halves)
- 1/3 cup dried cranberries

Combine all in a bowl and top with a lemon/lime dressing.

Lemon/Lime Dressing:

- 1/3 cup fresh lemon juice
- 1/3 cup fresh lime juice
- 1 tsp. Dijon mustard
- 1/3 cup extra virgin olive oil
- 1/2 tsp. honey or maple syrup
- 1/3 tsp. dried oregano
- Sea salt and black pepper to taste

SOUPS RECIPES

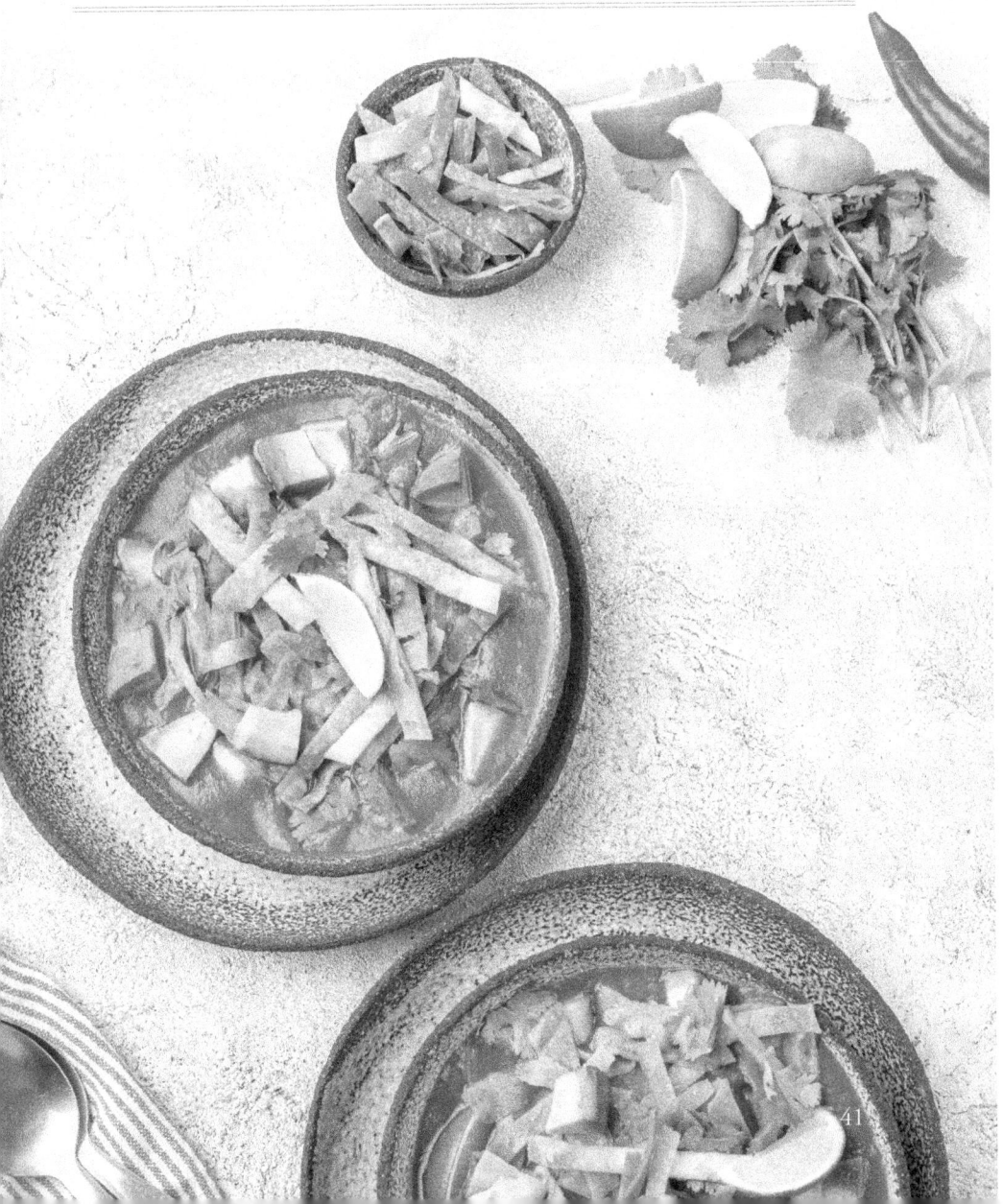

ENCHILADA SOUP

Ingredients:

- 1 Tbsp. olive oil
- 1 shallot onion, diced
- 2 red bell peppers, diced
- 2 jalapeño peppers (1 seeded and minced, 1 thinly sliced, optional)
- 1 tsp. ground cumin
- 2 tsps. garlic powder
- 1 tsp. kosher salt, plus more to taste
- 4 cups *Pacific* low-sodium vegetable broth
- 1 (15-oz.) can *Siete* red enchilada sauce
- 1 cup frozen or fresh corn
- 1 (15-oz.) can organic diced tomatoes
- 1 (15-oz.) can organic black beans, drained and rinsed
- 1 (15-oz.) can organic pinto beans, drained and rinsed
- 6 oz. tortilla chips - most are gluten-free, but check labels
- 1 cup shredded *Violife* Mexican cheese blend
- Black pepper, to taste
- *Violife* sour cream
- Sliced avocado, for topping

Directions:

In a large pot, heat the olive oil over medium-high heat. Add the onion, bell peppers, minced jalapeño, cumin, garlic powder, and salt. Cook, stirring, until the vegetables begin to soften and char in spots, 7 to 8 minutes. Add the broth, enchilada sauce, corn, tomatoes, black beans, and pinto beans. Bring to a boil over high heat, then reduce the heat to medium and simmer until the soup is thickened and reduced slightly, 10 to 12 minutes.

Meanwhile, preheat the broiler. Spread the tortilla chips in a single layer on a baking sheet and top with the cheese. Broil until the cheese is melted, 2 to 3 minutes, rotating the baking sheet as needed to avoid burning.

Season the soup with salt and pepper to taste. Divide among bowls and top with the chips, sour cream, avocado, and sliced jalapeño.

I'm big on Mexican foods. That's where this recipe came about. I was craving that Mexican spice and needing something that I could palate more without having that dairy and gluten. This hit the spot perfectly.

CHICKEN POT PIE SOUP

Ingredients:

- 4 Tbsp. salted butter (*Country Crock Plant Butter* for dairy and gluten-free)
- 3 stalks celery, finely diced
- 2 medium carrots, peeled and finely diced
- 2 medium onion, finely diced
- 2 tsp. chopped fresh thyme
- Pinch of turmeric
- Kosher salt and black pepper, to taste
- 1/4 cup *King Arthur* all-purpose gluten-free flour
- 1/2 cup white wine
- 6 cups chicken broth
- 3 cups shredded rotisserie chicken
- 1/4 cup chopped fresh parsley
- 1/2 cup *Let's Do Organic* heavy coconut cream

Directions:

Melt the butter in a large pot over medium heat. Add the celery, carrots, onion, and thyme. Season with the turmeric and a good pinch of salt and pepper. Stir and cook until the vegetables begin to soften, 3 to 4 minutes. Sprinkle the flour over the vegetables, and stir until combined, letting the flour cook for 1 to 2 minutes. While stirring, slowly pour in the wine and chicken broth. Add the chicken and parsley. Let the soup come to a boil and thicken slightly. Stir in the cream, and taste. Adjust seasonings as needed. Serve the soup and enjoy this delightful meal.

This will serve 4-6 people or give you leftovers for days. It can also be frozen to enjoy at a later date.

PASTA FAGIOLI SOUP

Ingredients:

- 1/2 pound Italian turkey sausage links, casings removed, crumbled
- 1 small shallot onion, chopped
- 1-1/2 tsps. avocado oil
- 1 garlic clove, minced
- 2 cups water
- 1 can (14-1/2 oz.) organic diced tomatoes, undrained
- 1 can (14-1/2 oz.) *Pacific* reduced-sodium chicken broth
- 3/4 cup uncooked *Jovial* elbow pasta, gluten-free
- 1/4 tsp. pepper
- 1 cup fresh spinach leaves, cut as desired
- 5 tsps. shredded *Violife* Parmesan cheese

Directions:

In a large saucepan, cook sausage over medium heat until no longer pink; drain, remove from pan, and set aside. In the same pan, saute onion in oil until tender. Add garlic; sauté 1 minute longer. Add the water, tomatoes, broth, elbow noodles, and pepper. Bring to a boil. Cook, uncovered, until noodles are tender, 8-10 minutes. Reduce heat to low; stir in sausage and spinach. Cook until spinach is wilted, 2-3 minutes. Garnish with cheese and serve.

EASY BISON SOUP

Ingredients:

- 1/2 pound ground bison
- 2 cups water
- 1 can (14-1/2 oz.) stewed tomatoes
- 1 pkg. (10 oz.) frozen organic mixed vegetables
- 1 can (8 oz.) tomato sauce
- 1 envelope onion soup mix, Lipton has a gluten-free mixture
- 1/2 tsp. sugar

Directions:

In a saucepan over medium heat, cook bison until no longer pink, breaking into crumbles; drain. Add the remaining ingredients; bring to a boil. Reduce heat; cover and simmer until vegetables are tender. It's ready to be served. Enjoy!

CREAMY CHICKEN SOUP

Ingredients:

- 2 cooked chicken breasts, shredded
- 2 Tbsp. olive oil
- 1 large shallot onion, diced
- 2 large carrots, diced
- 1 large celery stalk, diced
- 3 garlic cloves, minced
- 32 oz. *Pacific* chicken broth or stock
- 1 Tbsp. fresh chopped thyme
- 1 Tbsp. fresh chopped dill
- 1 Tbsp. fresh chopped parsley
- 1/2 Tbsp. fresh chopped cilantro
- 1 Tbsp. fresh chopped basil
- 1 can *Pacific* gluten-free cream of chicken soup
- 2 cups *Jovial* - Organic Brown Rice Pasta, fusilli
- kosher salt and fresh ground pepper to taste

Directions:

Combine ingredients in a medium size sauce pan, bring to a boil, then turn down and simmer till vegetables are tender.

Who doesn't just love a warm bowl of chicken soup? The broth alone supports the body in many ways. Helps support the respiratory system (which I needed all the help I could get) and gets things to open up so that you can breathe more comfortable. Having severe asthma and severe allergies that trigger my respiratory system, this soup has helped save me from breathing troubles in many ways and helped to ease the discomfort in my chest during attacks.

CHICKEN GINGER SOUP

Try to use as much fresh organic herbs as you can.

Ingredients:

- 2 Tbsp. olive oil
- 1 large shallot onion – chopped
- 4 large carrots – chopped
- 3 stalks celery – chopped
- 2 cups shredded cabbage
- Kosher salt and freshly ground black pepper, to taste
- 1 tsp. turmeric
- 1 tsp. onion powder
- 1/2 tsp. rosemary
- 1/2 tsp. thyme
- 3 cloves garlic – minced
- 4 Tbsp. ginger – minced
- 9-10 cups *Pacific* lower-sodium chicken broth
- 2.5 pounds chicken breast, cut into two-inch cubes
- 2 cups frozen peas or you can use fresh snap peas

Directions:

In a large stock pot over medium-high heat, add olive oil, and then the chopped onion, carrots, celery, and cabbage. Cook until slightly softened, about 6-7 minutes. Add the garlic, ginger, and seasonings – salt, pepper, turmeric, onion powder, rosemary, and thyme. Cook for a couple of minutes, stirring constantly. Then add the chicken broth and bring to a boil. Season the chicken breast with salt and add it to the pot over medium heat. Cook until done, about 15 minutes.

Remove chicken and set aside to cool slightly. Shred chicken with two forks, or add it to a standing mixer to shred. Add it back to the pot, along with the frozen peas. Continue simmering for about 10 minutes or until peas are warm. Check seasonings, and serve with some freshly ground black pepper. This will activate they turmeric in this soup.

My bodies inflammation markers were very high when I became ill but had no clue until the right tests where done that actually showed true numbers of how inflamed my body was. This is a great soup to make when the body is inflamed and you need to bring the levels down. It'll help reduce swelling, bloating and leave your body feeling refreshed, relaxed and ease your mind of worry.

TACO SOUP

Ingredients:

- 2 tsp. olive oil
- 1 1/4 lbs ground bison
- 1 medium shallot onion chopped (1 ½ cups)
- 2 cloves garlic, minced (2 tsp.)
- 1 jalapeno, seeded and finely chopped (optional)
- 2 (14.5 oz.) cans organic diced tomatoes with green chilies
- 1 (14 oz.) can *Pacific* low-sodium beef or vegetable broth
- 1 (8 oz.) can tomato sauce (*Muir Glen* and *Bionaturae* brands are both gluten-free)
- 1 Tbsp. chili powder
- 1 tsp. ground cumin
- 3/4 tsp. ground paprika
- 1/4 tsp. dried oregano
- 1 1/2 Tbsp. dry ranch dressing mix (See Notes for Recipe), or substitute with 1/3 cup chopped cilantro and 1 Tbsp. fresh lime juice
- Salt and freshly ground black pepper to taste
- 1 1/2 cups frozen or fresh corn
- 1 (14.5 oz.) can *Serious Bean Co.* black beans, drained and rinsed
- 1 (14.5 oz.) can *Eden* pinto beans, drained and rinsed
- Toppings: *Violife* Shredded Mexican blend cheese
- Chopped green or red onions
- Diced avocados
- *Fresh Gourmet Tri-color* corn tortilla strips

Directions:

Heat a large pot over medium-high heat drizzle lightly with oil. Add ground bison in with chopped onion, crumbling and stirring occasionally until browned. Add jalapeno and garlic, and saute 1 minute longer. Drain excess fat from bison mixture. Stir in tomatoes with chilies, beef or vegetable broth, tomato sauce, chili powder, cumin, paprika, oregano, ranch dressing mix, and season with salt and pepper to tastes. Cover pot with lid and simmer 30 minutes, stirring occasionally. Add in corn, black beans, and pinto beans and cook until heated through. Add 1/2 cup water to thin soup if desired. Stir in cilantro and lime if using. Serve warm finished with desired toppings.

NOTES FOR TACO SOUP:

How to make a dairy-free and gluten-free dry ranch mix.

Produce

- 1/2 tsp. chives, dried
- 1/2 tsp. dill, dried
- 1/2 tsp. garlic powder
- 1/2 tsp. onion powder
- 1/2 tsp. parsley, dried

Canned Goods

- 1/2 cup coconut milk, full fat

Condiments

- 1/2 cup vegan mayo

Baking Spices

- 1/2 tsp. pepper
- 1/2 tsp. salt

Vinegars

- 1 tsp. apple cider vinegar

Loving that Mexican style soup but being allergic to most of the ingredients in your normal taco soup, I decided (with the suggestion of Niki) to create this dairy and gluten-free taco soup made with ground bison 'cus, yep, I can't have that beef either. Since bison has a stronger taste, this turned out wonderful and gave me a different feeling for bison meat. It's a taco soup that will surprise you with a wonderful flavor and you'll want to try more recipes with bison in them.

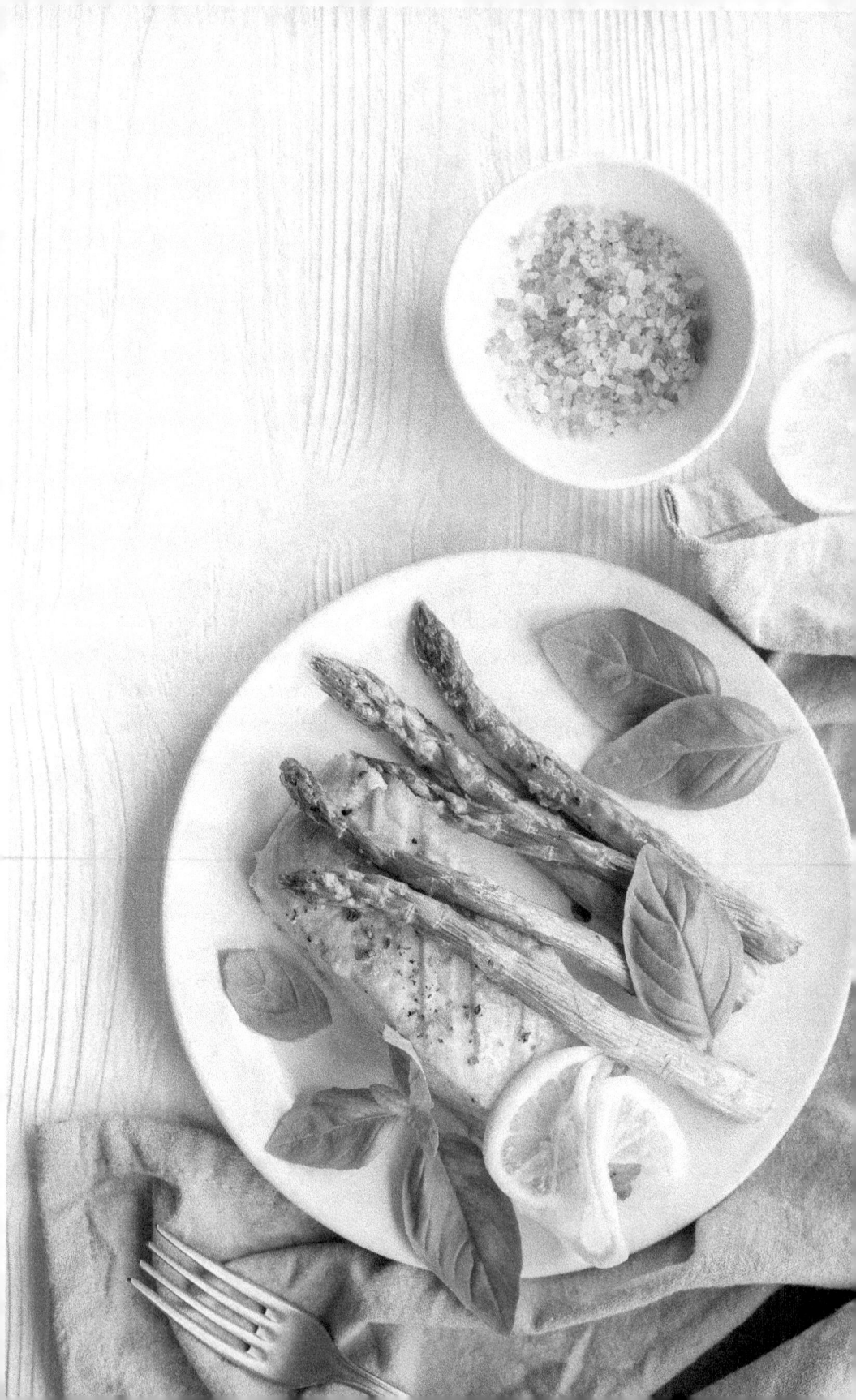

ENTREES

I have prepared a variety of items for Adam and Heidi, ranging from meals to smoothies and desserts. I am pleased to note that they have enjoyed everything. As my medical care team through Nutrition IV services at IV Nutrition-St. Joseph, MO, they have provided exceptional care. Our friendship extends beyond the professional realm, as they have treated me and my children with kindness and compassion, making their role in my recovery a truly blessed experience.

What they have to say:

"Your food made dinner easier. We all enjoyed it. We've been so touched by everyone's kindness. It really helps, thank you!"
"Green juice was delicious! Thanks!"
"Felt like we were eating a fancy dessert!"
"We just broke out the blueberry smoothie! Delicious! Thank you!"
"The smoothies were delicious! All of the food was amazing! Thank you again!!"
—Adam and Heidi Merritt

SMOTHERED SPINACH CHICKEN

Ingredients:

- 1 pkg. of chicken tenders, diced
- 1 cup spinach, chopped
- 1/4 diced yellow, red, orange, green peppers
- 1/4 shallot onion
- 2 cloves garlic, minced
- 1 Tbsp. oregano
- 1 Tbsp. Italian seasoning
- 1 tsp. paprika or cayenne pepper
- 1 can of gluten-free cream of mushroom soup (Pacific Foods Brand)

Directions:

In a skillet, along with garlic, peppers and onion, cook chicken until done.

Sauce: In a sauce pan on medium to low heat, prepare cream of mushroom soup, spinach, oregano, Italian seasoning, and paprika or cayenne pepper. Pour sauce over the chicken and serve. Add gluten-free pasta for an additional dish!

CHICKEN WITH GARLIC PARMESAN RICE

Ingredients:

- 2 Tbsps. olive oil
- 1/2 cup (one stick) *Violife* butter
- 1 pound chicken tenders
- 1/2 tsp. garlic powder
- 2 Tbsps. minced garlic
- 1 tsp. salt, divided in half
- 1/4 tsp. red pepper flakes
- 1 1/2 cup white rice, (gluten-free, uncooked)
- 1/2 cup dry white wine, (such as Pinot Grigio)
- 1/2 cup Parmesan cheese, (grated or shredded)
- 3 cups chicken broth
- Salt and pepper to taste

Directions:

In a large skillet, heat the olive oil over medium heat. In the meantime, season the chicken with salt, pepper, and garlic powder. Place the chicken into the skillet and sear until browned and completely cooked. Set aside when done.

In the same skillet, place the butter, garlic, pepper flakes, and 1/2 tsp. of salt. Saute over medium heat for a few minutes. Adjust the heat to medium-high, then pour in the white wine. Cook for approximately 5 minutes, stirring constantly. Reserve 3 Tbsps. of the pan sauce for later.

In the remaining butter sauce in the skillet, add the uncooked rice. Stir well. Pour in the chicken broth and season with the rest of the half tsp. of salt. Bring everything to a low boil. Once boiling, adjust the heat to medium-low. Put the lid on and simmer for about 20 minutes or until the rice is tender, stirring often.

Sprinkle on the Parmesan cheese and arrange the chicken tenders. Replace the lid and take the skillet off the heat. Allow the dish to stand for about 5 minutes. Before serving, drizzle the reserved pan sauce on top of the chicken. Garnish with some parsley. Enjoy!

VEGGIE SWEET N' SOUR CHICKEN

Ingredients:

- 1 pkg organic chicken tenders, diced/cubed
- 1/4 cup of the following items:
  green pepper
  red pepper
  yellow pepper
  orange pepper
  shallot onion
- 2 cloves garlic
- 1/4 cup raw honey
- 1/2 cup shredded zucchini
- 1/2 cup peas
- Salt and pepper to taste

Directions:

Cook veggies and peppers in a spread pan til then are softened, then combine after draining chicken and add your sweet n' sour sauce—about a half cup. Serve over rice or pasta.

HOMEMADE CHICKEN HELPER MEAL

Ingredients:

- 2-4 chicken breasts- shredded
- 1 Jar Rao's Homemade Marinara Sauce
- 1 Garlic Alfredo sauce (*Primal Kitchen* is dairy free & gluten-free)
- 2 Tbsps. garlic powder
- 1/3 cup red onion, diced
- 1/2 shallot onion, diced
- 1 Tbsp. Italian seasoning
- 1 Tbsp. drained parsley
- 1/2 container of *Kite Hill* ricotta cheese
- 1/2 cup chopped spinach and kale
- 1 box Jovial Gluten-Free Farfalle
- red pepper, yellow pepper, orange pepper (as much as desired or optional)
- Salt and pepper to taste

Directions:

Cook chicken breasts in 1 cup of chicken broth for 25-30 minutes. Shred with a fork.

In a separate dish, mix a jar of *Rao's* homemade marinara sauce and garlic alfredo sauce, and cook pasta until tender. Then mix in the remaining ingredients, except the spinach and kale, and cook until ricotta cheese is melted down. When ready, mix in the shredded chicken, top with spinach and kale, and cook 5 minutes longer before serving.

The taste will leave you craving more. Healthy, high in protein, and good source of fiber, it will keep you full for much longer.

HOMEMADE BISON HELPER MEAL

Ingredients:

- 1 lb. ground bison
- 1 Jar Rao's Homemade Marinara Sauce
- 1 Garlic Alfredo sauce (*Primal Kitchen* is dairy free & gluten-free)
- 2 Tbsps. garlic powder
- 1/3 cup red onion, diced
- 1/2 shallot onion, diced
- 1 Tbsp. Italian seasoning
- 1 Tbsp. drained parsley
- 1/2 container of *Kite Hill* ricotta cheese
- 1/2 cup chopped spinach and kale
- 1 box *Jovial* Gluten-Free Farfalle
- red pepper, yellow pepper, orange pepper (as much as desired or optional)
- Salt and pepper to taste

Directions:

Cook bison until done.

In a separate dish, mix a jar of *Rao's* homemade marinara sauce and garlic Alfredo sauce, and cook pasta until tender. Then mix in the remaining ingredients, except the spinach and kale, and cook until ricotta cheese is melted down. When ready, mix in the ground bison, top with spinach and kale, and cook 5 minutes longer before serving.

The taste will leave you craving more, and no one will be able to tell it's bison. Healthy, high protein, and a good source of fiber. It will keep you full for longer. Great for family gatherings or celebrations.

CRISPY MUSHROOM TOAST WITH RICOTTA

Ingredients:

- 1 Tbsp. olive oil
- 8 oz. mixed mushrooms (such as shiitake, cremini, and oyster), trimmed and sliced
- 1/4 cup *Kite Hill* ricotta cheese
- 2 Tbsps. unsalted *Violife* butter, room temperature
- 4 slices of country-style bread, toasted
- Kosher salt to taste
- Freshly ground black pepper to taste
- Finely grated Parmesan, for serving
- Chopped fresh chives, for serving

Directions:

In a large skillet, heat the olive oil over medium-high heat. Add the mixed mushrooms and season with salt and pepper. Cook, stirring occasionally, until the mushrooms are golden brown and crispy, about 8-10 minutes. Remove from heat and set aside.

In a small bowl, mix the ricotta cheese and unsalted butter until well combined. Spread the ricotta mixture evenly onto the toasted slices of country-style bread. Top each slice of bread with a generous amount of the crispy mushrooms. Sprinkle finely grated Parmesan over the mushrooms and garnish with chopped fresh chives. Serve the crispy mushroom toast with ricotta immediately, while warm, and enjoy the delightful crunch and creamy texture!

ITALIAN CHICKEN ZUCCHINI PIZZA

Ingredients:

- 1 Zucchini, diced into cubes
- 1 pkg. chicken tenders or breast, cooked & shredded
- 1/2 cup Italian seasoning
- 1/4 cup vary of chopped bell peppers
- 1/4 cup shallot onion
- 1/4 cup chopped bella mushrooms
- 3 cloves diced garlic
- 1 16-oz. pizza sauce
- 1/2 cup dairy & gluten-free mozzarella cheese

Directions:

Mix everything together besides cheese and pizza sauce. Cook in skillet on stove. When cooked, mix in baking dish with pizza sauce & cheese. Bake at 425° for 20 mins. Serve with shake Parmesan cheese that's dairy and gluten-free.

SWEET & SMOKY JALAPEÑO STUFF CHICKEN

Ingredients:

- 4 chicken breast, cut in half but not all the way through, making a pocket
- 2 jalapeños sliced in half, cleaned
- Panko gluten-free sweet and smoky bread crumbs

Stuffing mixture:

- 1/4 *Violife* cream cheese
- 1/4 *Kite Rite* ricotta cheese
- 1/4 green pepper, minced
- 1/4 red pepper, minced
- 1/4 yellow pepper, minced
- 1/4 orange pepper, minced
- 1/2 shallot onion, minced
- 4 garlic cloves, minced
- 1/3 cup *Violife* mozzarella cheese

Directions:

Mix stuffing ingredients together. Stuff jalapeño halves and place in pocket of chicken breast. Roll chicken breast in sweet and smoky bread crumbs. Place in baking dish and bake at 425° for 40 minutes.

"If you're looking for a dish that delivers pure comfort with a gourmet twist, look no further than this grilled chicken stuffed with cream cheese—it's nothing short of mouthwatering perfection. The chicken is juicy and tender, kissed by the smoky char of the grill, and bursting with a rich, creamy center. The cream cheese melts into every bite, turning the inside into a decadent surprise of velvety smoothness, often blended with herbs, garlic, or a hint of spice to elevate the flavor. Each forkful is a harmony of savory, smoky, and creamy—simple yet unforgettable. It's the kind of meal that makes you pause, close your eyes, and savor every second. A true showstopper on the plate."

—Courtney Chamberlain

CHICKEN BACON RANCH ROLL-UPS

Ingredients:

- 2/3 cups of *Violife* mozzarella cheese
- 1 1/2 cups cooked chicken, shredded
- 1/4 cup cooked bacon (2-3 slices)
- 1 Tbsp. dairy-free ranch dressing
- 1 tsp. finely sliced green onion
- 1 pkg. gluten-free tortillas

Directions:

Combine shredded chicken, cooked bacon, ranch dressing, and green onions in a bowl. Set aside.

Preheat the oven to 350°F and line a large baking sheet with a silicone baking mat. Arrange the tortillas and line with mozzarella on the silicone baking mat. Bake for 5-7 minutes or until the cheese is semi melted. Remove from the oven and let cool for about a minute, cool enough to handle.

Spread the chicken, bacon, & ranch mixture along one edge of each mozzarella tortilla. Roll up tightly with the seam side down. Once finished, bake for another 3 minutes or until tortilla is browned.

STUFFED JALAPEÑO TURKEY BREAST

Ingredients:

- 4 small boneless turkey breasts (about 5 oz. each)
- 4 large jalapeño peppers, sliced in half and cleaned free of seeds
- 4 ounces *Violife* cream cheese, chilled
- 2 Tbsps. *Kite Hill* ricotta alternative, dairy free
- Celtic salt and freshly ground black pepper to taste
- 1/2 cup Colby Jack cheese (dairy and gluten-free)
- 1/4 Tbsp. oregano
- 1/4 Tbsp. Italian seasoning
- 1/4 Tbsp. garlic powder or 3 cloves, minced
- 20 slices bacon or turkey bacon (about 1 1/2 pounds), optional

Directions:

Cut the turkey breast down the middle but not slicing completely through. Mix cream cheese, celtic salt, freshly ground pepper, colby jack cheese, ricotta, oregano, Italian seasoning, and garlic in a bowl. Fill the inside of the sliced jalapeños with your mixture, then place it in the sliced part of the turkey breast. Fold back over and wrap with turkey bacon or close and hold it together with toothpicks. Place in a glass dish and bake for 45 minutes at 425° or place in an air fryer.

Hint: The air fryer might bring the cooking time down by 10/15 minutes, but cook until turkey is done.

BISON MEATLOAF DISH

Ingredients:

- 1lb Bison
- 1 zucchini, shredded
- 1 egg
- 1 cup carrots, shredded
- 4 stalks celery, diced
- 1/2 cup *4c* brand gluten-free bread crumbs
- 1/4 cup bell peppers, chopped (optional)
- 1/4 shallot onion
- 1/4 cup bella mushrooms, chopped
- 3 cloves garlic, diced
- 1/2 cup *Violife* dairy & gluten-free mozzarella cheese or cheese of choice
- 1/4 cup parsley for topping after baked

Directions:

Mix everything together. Make into a loaf and bake at 425° for 35 to 40 minutes. Top with *Sweet Baby Ray's* original BBQ sauce or Dijon mustard, then bake for 10 more minutes. Add parsley.

TERIYAKI CHICKEN LETTUCE WRAPS

Ingredients:

- 1 pound boneless, skinless chicken breasts, diced
- 1/4 cup teriyaki sauce
- 2 Tbsps. honey
- 2 cloves garlic, minced
- 1 tsp. fresh ginger, grated
- 1 Tbsp. sesame oil
- 1 Tbsp. cornstarch
- 2 Tbsps. water
- 1 Tbsp. avocado oil
- 1 red bell pepper, diced
- 1/2 cup carrots, shredded
- 1/4 cup green onions, chopped
- 1/4 cup cilantro, chopped
- Butter lettuce leaves, for serving
- Sesame seeds, for garnish

Directions:

In a bowl, whisk together the Teriyaki sauce, honey, minced garlic, grated ginger, and sesame oil. In a separate small bowl, mix together the cornstarch and water to create a slurry.

Heat avocado oil in a large skillet over medium-high heat. Add diced chicken and cook until browned and cooked through. Pour the teriyaki sauce over the chicken in the skillet. Stir to coat evenly. Add the diced red bell pepper and shredded carrots to the skillet. Cook for an additional 2-3 minutes until vegetables are tender-crisp. Stir in the cornstarch slurry and cook until the sauce thickens, about 1-2 minutes. Remove from heat and stir in chopped green onions and cilantro.

To serve, spoon the chicken mixture into butter lettuce leaves. Garnish with sesame seeds. Enjoy.

GOBBLER POPPERS

Ingredients:

- 2 8-oz. pkgs. *Violife* cream cheese, softened
- 2 cups *Violife* cheddar cheese, shredded
- 10 jalapeño peppers, halved and seeded
- 1 12-oz pkg. turkey bacon

Directions:

Preheat the oven to 350°.

Mix together cream cheese and cheddar cheese in a large bowl until well combined. Spread cheese mixture into the center of each jalapeño half.

Cut bacon slices in half crosswise. Wrap 1 bacon strip around the center of each jalapeño half.

Place wrapped jalapeños on a nonstick baking sheet. Bake in the preheated oven until bacon is cooked and jalapeños are slightly tender, 10 to 15 minutes.

Tips: If you like your bacon extra crispy, I suggest using precooked turkey bacon. You can add some jalapeño seeds to the cream cheese mixture for an extra kick.

"Golden, crispy, and irresistibly indulgent—jalapeño poppers are the ultimate bite-sized delight. Each fresh, green jalapeño is sliced and hollowed just enough to cradle a creamy, tangy filling of rich cream cheese and sharp cheddar. The pepper's natural heat mingles perfectly with the cool, velvety center, creating a bold contrast in every bite. Many are wrapped in smoky bacon, adding a savory, salty finish that crisps up beautifully in the oven. They're warm, spicy, creamy, and just the right amount of bold—perfect for sharing, but hard to resist keeping all to yourself."

—Courtney Chamberlain

HOMEMADE SLOPPY JOE

Ingredients:

- 2 lbs. hamburger or bison
- 1 green pepper diced
- 1 small shallot onion diced

Sauce:

- 2 cups ketchup
- 3 Tbsps. brown sugar
- 3 Tbsps. yellow mustard
- 2 Tbsps. Worcestershire sauce
- 1 Tbsp. pepper
- 1 Tbsp. garlic powder

Directions:

Brown hamburger with veggies. Drain. Cook sauce ingredients on low for 30 min. and add to cooked meat and veggie mixture.

GARLIC HONEY SALMON WITH ASPARAGUS

Ingredients:

- 4 salmon fillets (about 6 ounces each)
- 4 Tbsps. *Violife* butter, melted
- 4 cloves garlic, minced
- 3 Tbsps. honey
- 2 Tbsps. Dijon mustard
- 2 Tbsps. fresh parsley, chopped
- 1 Tbsp. lemon juice
- 4 lemon slices
- 5 sticks of asparagus per foil
- Salt and pepper, to taste

Directions:

Preheat your oven to 375°F (190°C).

Place each salmon fillet on a piece of aluminum foil large enough to fold over and seal. Season each fillet with salt and pepper.

In a bowl, mix together melted butter, minced garlic, honey, and Dijon mustard. Spoon the garlic butter mixture over the salmon fillets evenly. Sprinkle chopped parsley on top and add lemon slices if desired along with asparagus. Fold the foil over the salmon and seal to create a packet.

Bake for 15-20 minutes, or until salmon is cooked through and flakes easily with a fork. Serve hot, garnished with additional fresh parsley and lemon slices.

GARLIC BUTTER CHICKEN BITES WITH LEMON ASPARAGUS

Ingredients:

- 3-4 boneless, skinless chicken breasts, cut into bite-sized chunks
- 2 bunches of asparagus, rinsed and trimmed
- 1/2 cup *Violife* butter, softened
- 1 tsp. olive oil
- 2 tsps. garlic, minced
- 1 tsp. Italian seasoning
- 1 Tbsp. hot sauce, optional
- 1/2 cup low-sodium chicken broth (or white wine)
- Juice of 1/2 lemon
- 1 Tbsp. minced parsley
- Crushed red chili pepper flakes, optional
- Slices of lemon, for garnish

For the chicken seasoning:

- 2 tsps. salt
- 1 tsp. fresh cracked black pepper
- 2 tsps. onion powder

Directions:

Slice chicken breasts into bite-sized chunks and season with salt, pepper, and onion powder. Let sit in a shallow plate while you prepare the asparagus.

Wash and trim the ends of the asparagus, then blanch them in boiling water for 2 minutes. Soak in ice water to stop the asparagus from cooking further. This allows the asparagus to cook faster and more evenly in the skillet. (You can skip this step if you have very thin asparagus.) Drain and set aside.

Heat half of the butter and the olive oil in a large skillet over medium-low heat. Gently stir-fry the chicken bites on all sides until golden brown. Lower the heat and add 1 tsp. minced garlic and Italian seasoning. Stir and cook with chicken bites until fragrant. Remove the chicken bites from the skillet and set aside on a plate. (You might have to work in batches to avoid crowding the pan and have steamed chicken bites instead of browned.)

In the same skillet, over medium-high, add minced garlic and then deglaze with chicken broth (or wine). Bring to a simmer and allow to reduce to half the volume. Add remaining butter, lemon juice, hot sauce, parsley. Give a quick stir to combine. Add the blanched asparagus and toss for 2 minutes to cook it up. Add the sauteed chicken bites back to the pan and stir for another minute to reheat.

BACON GUACAMOLE GRILLED CHEESE SANDWICH

Ingredients:

- 1 Tbsp. salted butter, room temperature
- 2 slices sour dough bread (gluten-free)
- 1/2 cup *Violife* cheddar cheese, shredded (or 2 slices), room temperature
- 2 Tbsps. guacamole, room temperature
- 2 slices turkey bacon, cooked and crumbled (optional)
- 1 Tbsp. tortilla chips, crumbled (optional)

Directions:

Butter one side of each slice of bread. Sprinkle half of the cheese onto the unbuttered side of one slice of bread followed by the guacamole, bacon, tortilla chips, the remaining cheese and finally top with the remaining slice of bread with the buttered side up. Grill in a preheated pan over medium heat until golden brown on both sides and the cheese has melted, about 2-4 minutes per side.

GREEN SMOTHERED CHICKEN

Ingredients:

- 4 chicken breast, diced/cubed
- 1/2 cup spinach
- 1/4 cup kale
- 1/2 zucchini, sliced
- 1 can cream of chicken (gluten-free)
- 3 garlic cloves or 2 Tbsps. minced garlic
- 1/4 shallot onion
- 4 oz. chicken broth
- 3 Tbsps. garlic herb seasoning
- Salt and pepper to taste

Directions:

Mix all ingredients except chicken together in a blender and then smother over chicken in oven-safe dish. Bake for 35 minutes at 425° or steam on low heat on the stove for 45 minutes. Remove chicken from mixture and serve with your favorite sides, or gluten-free rice or pasta.

GARLIC PARMESAN CHICKEN SKEWERS

Ingredients:

- 2 lbs. chicken tenders, thighs or breast (or turkey breast or skewers)
- 2 Tbsps. olive oil
- Mushrooms, cut in pieces
- Onions, cut in pieces
- Bell peppers, cut in pieces
- Parmesan cheese (optional)

Garlic Parmesan Butter Sauce:

- 1 stick *Violife* butter
- 8-10 cloves garlic, minced

Directions:

Cut chicken into squares. Marinade in butter sauce for 30 minutes. Put on skewer sticks alternating with chunks of mushroom, onion, and pepper. Add grated Parmesan cheese after cooked to top it off.

VEGGIE CHICKEN OR TURKEY DISH

Ingredients:

- 2-3 chicken or turkey breasts, cubed
- 3-5 small to medium potatoes, cubed
- 2 cups of fresh green beans or broccoli (I used 1 1/2 cups of green beans)
- 1 pkg. dry Italian dressing mix
- 1 melted stick of *Violife* butter

Directions:

Place chicken, potatoes and beans in pan. Sprinkle Italian pack over everything, then drizzle the butter over top. Cover with foil and bake at 350 for an hour and 10 minutes.

STUFFED POBLANO PEPPERS

Ingredients:

- 6 large poblano peppers
- 1 lb. ground beef or bison
- 1 shallot onion, diced
- 2 cloves garlic, minced
- 2 tsps. chili powder
- 1 tsp. ground cumin
- 1 cup cooked brown rice
- 1 Cup chopped celery
- 1 cup black beans, rinsed and drained
- 1 14.5-ounce fire-roasted tomatoes, diced
- Celtic salt and freshly-ground black pepper to taste
- 1 1/2 cups shredded *Violife* Mexican blend cheese or Monterey Jack Cheese
- 1/4 cup chopped cilantro

Directions:

Preheat oven to 375°.

Cut 1/4-1/3 off the poblano peppers, lengthwise. Remove the veins and seeds. Place the peppers, cut side up, on a baking sheet covered in parchment paper and bake for 12-15 minutes or until somewhat soft.

Remove them from the oven and carefully turn them over to drain any excess moisture. Caution: they will be very hot.

Meanwhile, brown the meat in a large skillet over medium heat. About halfway through the browning process, add the onion and cook until the meat is browned and the onion is soft. Drain any excess grease from the pan. Turn the heat to low. Add the garlic, chili powder, and ground cumin. Cook for 1 minute while stirring constantly. Stir in the cooked rice, celery, black beans, and fire roasted tomatoes. Simmer for a few minutes over low heat. If the mixture becomes too thick, add 2 Tbsps. of beef broth, chicken broth or water. Season with Celtic salt and fresh ground black pepper. Remove the mixture from the heat and let it cool for a few minutes. Stir in 1 cup of cheese and 2-3 Tbsps. chopped cilantro.

Spoon the mixture into the poblano peppers and top with the remaining cheese. Return the stuffed peppers to the oven and bake for 10-15 minutes or until the cheese is melted and the peppers are heated through. Sprinkle with the remaining chopped cilantro.

Notes: For best results, buy the largest poblano pepper you can find. Choose large, firm peppers without blemishes or any sign of decay. Slice the top 1/4-1/3 of the pepper lengthwise above the stem. You can use a small paring knife to help so you have a large pocket left for the stuffing. Prepare the stuffing up to a day in advance. Garnish with enchilada sauce, sour cream, or chopped cilantro.

CHICKEN AND AVOCADO ENCHILADAS IN CREAMY AVOCADO SAUCE

Ingredients:

- 2 cups cooked chicken, shredded
- 2 ripe avocados, peeled, pitted, and diced
- 1 cup shredded *Violife* Monterey Jack cheese
- 1/4 cup chopped fresh cilantro
- 1/4 cup chopped green onions
- 1/2 tsp. ground cumin
- 1/2 tsp. chili powder
- Salt and pepper, to taste
- 10 small flour tortillas
- 2 cups enchilada sauce
- 1/2 cup *Violife* sour cream
- 1/4 cup chopped fresh cilantro, for garnish
- Lime wedges, for serving

Directions:

Preheat oven to 375°.

In a large mixing bowl, combine the cooked chicken, diced avocado, shredded Monterey Jack cheese, chopped cilantro, chopped green onions, ground cumin, chili powder, salt, and pepper. Mix until well combined.

Grease a 9x13-inch baking dish. Warm the flour tortillas in the microwave for about 20-30 seconds to make them pliable. Spoon the chicken and avocado mixture evenly onto each tortilla, then roll them up and place them seam-side down in the prepared baking dish. Pour the enchilada sauce over the top of the rolled enchiladas, making sure to cover them evenly. Bake in the preheated oven for 20-25 minutes, or until the enchiladas are heated through and the sauce is bubbly. Remove from the oven and let cool for a few minutes before serving. Drizzle the enchiladas with sour cream and sprinkle with chopped cilantro. Serve with lime wedges on the side.

SPINACH GARLIC MEATBALLS STUFFED WITH MOZZARELLA

Ingredients:

- 8 oz. baby spinach, fresh
- 3 cloves garlic, finely chopped
- 1-2 Tbsps. olive oil

Meatballs:

- 2 pound ground bison
- 1 pound ground pork
- 2 1/4 cups gluten-free bread crumbs
- 3 eggs (use 4 if eggs are small)
- Splash of Almond milk
- 4 garlic cloves, finely chopped
- 1/2 cup *Violife* Parmesan cheese
- Salt and pepper to taste
- 2 Tbsps. olive oil
- *Violife* mozzarella cheese
- 1 jar Prego gluten-free marinara sauce

Directions:

Heat 1-2 Tbsps. olive oil in a skillet and add baby spinach. Toss to coat and allow it to wilt. Add finely chopped garlic and sauté for a minute or two until fragrant. Remove the spinach from the skillet, chop it into small pieces, and let it cool.

Preheat oven to 350°F (175°C). In a large mixing bowl, combine ground bison, ground pork, bread crumbs, eggs, Almond milk, finely chopped garlic, Parmesan cheese, salt, pepper, and the cooled spinach/garlic mixture. Mix well. Roll the meat mixture into meatballs and stuff each one with a small amount of mozzarella cheese.

Heat 2 Tbsps. olive oil in skillet and pan-fry the meatballs until the outsides are golden brown. Add dollops of marinara sauce to the bottom of the skillet, as much or as little as you prefer. Remove from skillet and place in baking dish to the preheated oven. Bake for about 20-25 minutes or until the meatballs reach an internal temperature of 165°F (74°C). Serve the meatballs over pasta, and enjoy!

CHICKEN OR TURKEY BREAST STUFFIN'

Ingredients:

- 2-4 chicken or turkey breasts
- 3 ounces frozen chopped spinach, thawed and excess liquid squeezed out
- 3 cloves garlic, minced
- 3/4 cup *Kite Hill* ricotta cheese
- 1/4 cup shredded *Violife* Parmesan cheese
- 1/3 of *Violife* mozzarella cheese
- 1 1/2 tsp. garlic powder
- 1/4 shallot, minced
- Celtic salt and pepper to taste

Directions:

Preheat oven to 375°.

Slice chicken or turkey breast down the middle, not slicing all the way through. Pack some stuffing between the slices. Fold back together, place in glass baking dish and bake for 40 minutes.

Hint: You can also slice jalapeno's in half and stuff them, then lay them in the middle of your sliced chicken or turkey breast for a little extra kick and flavor.

CREAMY GARLIC PARMESAN MUSHROOMS

Ingredients:

- 2 Tbsps. *VitaLife* butter (or any dairy-free)
- 1 Tbsp. olive oil
- 8 ounces bella mushrooms, whole or sliced to preference
- 2 cloves garlic, minced
- 1/2 cup *Silk* dairy-free heavy cream
- 1/4 cup *Violife* Parmesan cheese, grated
- 2 ounces *Violife* cream cheese, softened
- 1 tsp. dried Italian seasoning
- 1/2 tsp. salt
- 1/4 tsp. pepper
- Fresh chopped parsley for garnish

Directions:

In a medium-sized skillet over medium-high heat, add the butter and olive oil. Add the mushrooms and garlic, and saute until tender. Add the heavy cream, Parmesan cheese, cream cheese, Italian seasoning, salt, and pepper. Stir over heat until the sauce is bubbly and smooth. Serve immediately and garnish with fresh parsley.

TERIYAKI CHICKEN PAN

Ingredients:

- 4 boneless, skinless chicken breasts
- 1 cup pineapple chunks
- 1 red bell pepper, diced
- 1 green bell pepper, diced
- 1 Shallot onion, diced
- 1/4 cup teriyaki sauce
- 1/4 cup raw honey
- 2 Tbsps. olive oil
- 2 cloves garlic, minced
- 1 tsp. ground ginger
- Salt and pepper to taste
- Cooked rice, for serving

Directions:

Preheat your oven to 400° and grease a large baking sheet.

In a small bowl, whisk together the soy sauce, honey, olive oil, minced garlic, ground ginger, salt, and pepper. Place the chicken breasts in the center of the prepared baking sheet, and arrange the pineapple chunks, diced bell peppers, and diced red onion around the chicken. Pour the soy sauce mixture over the chicken and vegetables, making sure everything is evenly coated. Bake in the preheated oven for 20-25 minutes, or until the chicken is cooked through and the vegetables are tender, flipping the chicken halfway through cooking. Remove from the oven and let it rest for a few minutes. Serve the Hawaiian chicken and vegetables over cooked rice. Enjoy your delicious Hawaiian chicken sheet pan dinner!

SLOW COOKER BBQ HONEY GARLIC CHICKEN

Ingredients:

Honey Garlic Sauce:

- 1/3 cup honey
- 1 Tbsp. garlic, minced
- 1/2 cup tamari sauce
- 1/4 cup BBQ sauce
- 1 tsp. dried oregano

Crockpot Chicken and Vegetables:

- 2 pounds chicken thighs, bone-in, skin-on
- 1 pound baby red potatoes
- 1 pound carrots, peeled
- 1 cup Shallot onions, chopped
- 1 pound green beans, trimmed
- Salt and pepper to taste
- Fresh parsley, chopped, for serving (optional)

Directions:

In a small bowl, whisk together honey, garlic, tamari sauce, oregano and BBQ sauce. Add the chicken thighs, potatoes, carrots and onions to a 4-6 quart slow cooker. Pour the honey garlic sauce mixture evenly on top. Cover the slow cooker and seal the lid. Cook on a LOW setting for 6-8 hours or on HIGH for 3-3 1/2 hours (see note).

About 20 minutes before serving, add the green beans to the slow cooker and optional cornstarch slurry to the sauce. Re-seal the lid and cook for 15-20 minutes more until the green beans are tender and the sauce is starting to thicken. Remove the chicken and vegetables to serving plates using a slotted spoon.

Optional: Broil the chicken thighs for 2-3 minutes to brown the skin. Drizzle sauce on top of chicken and vegetables. Garnish with optional minced parsley.

CHEESY GARLIC ZUCCHINI STEAKS

Ingredients:

- 2 medium zucchini Kosher salt
- 4 cloves garlic, finely chopped or grated
- 1/4 tsp. crushed red pepper flakes, plus more for serving
- 4 Tbsps. extra-virgin olive oil, divided
- 2 oz. *Violife* mozzarella, shredded
- 1 oz. *Violife* Parmesan, finely shredded (about 1/2 cup)
- 2 Tbsps. fresh basil, torn

Directions:

Place a rack in center of oven, and preheat to 425°.

Using a sharp knife, slice each zucchini in half lengthwise, yielding 4 "steaks." Score flesh side of each steak 1/4" deep diagonally at 1/2" intervals. Rotate steaks 90° and score diagonally again to create a crosshatch pattern. Season steaks on scored sides with 1 tsp. salt. Let sit to allow zucchini to release moisture, about 15 minutes.

In a large skillet over medium heat, cook garlic, red pepper flakes, and 2 Tbsps. olive oil, stirring, until garlic is fragrant – 1 to 2 minutes. Scrape garlic oil into a small bowl. In same skillet over medium-high heat, heat 1 Tbsp. olive oil. Pat zucchini dry. Arrange 2 halves flesh side down in skillet and cook until golden brown on the bottom – 2 to 3 minutes. Transfer to a baking sheet flesh side up. Repeat with remaining zucchini and 1 Tbsp. olive oil. Brush steaks with garlic oil. Bake zucchini until tender in the center – 8 to 10 minutes. Top with mozzarella and Parmesan. Heat broiler on high. Broil, watching closely, until cheese is melted and browned – 2 to 3 minutes. Transfer zucchini to a platter. Top with basil and more red pepper flakes.

PINEAPPLE CHICKEN AND RICE

Ingredients:

- 1 pound chicken breast, cubed
- 1 cup pineapple, cubed
- 1 Tbsp. olive oil
- 1 onion, chopped
- 2 cloves garlic, minced
- 1 red bell pepper, diced
- 1 cup brown rice
- 2 cups chicken broth
- 1 Tbsp. tamari sauce
- 1 tsp. ginger, grated
- Salt and pepper to taste
- 1/4 cup green onions, sliced
- 1 Tbsp. sesame seeds

Directions:

In a large skillet, heat the olive oil over medium heat. Add the chicken cubes and cook until golden brown and cooked through. Remove the chicken and set aside.

In the same skillet, add the onion, garlic, and red bell pepper. Cook until the vegetables are softened. Add the pineapple and cook for an additional 2 minutes. Stir in the jasmine rice, chicken broth, soy sauce, ginger, salt, and pepper. Bring to a boil. Reduce the heat to low, cover, and simmer for 18-20 minutes, or until the rice is cooked through.

Return the chicken to the skillet, mix well, and heat through. Serve garnished with green onions and sesame seeds.

GARLIC MUSHROOMS CAULIFLOWER SKILLET

Ingredients:

- 4 Tbsps. unsalted butter (*Vitalife* for dairy free or any)
- 1 Tbsp. pure olive oil
- 1/2 organic Shallot onion, chopped (about 1/2 cup)
- 1/2 head organic cauliflower, cut into florets (about 2 cups)
- 1 pound (500 g) organic Bella mushrooms, cleaned (about 4 cups)
- 2 Tbsps. organic vegetable stock
- 1 tsp. fresh organic thyme leaves, chopped
- 2 Tbsps. fresh organic parsley, chopped
- 4 cloves organic garlic, minced
- 1/4 cup *Violife* mozzarella if desired
- 1/2 tsp. salt and pepper, or to taste

Directions:

Heat the butter and oil in a large skillet over medium-high heat. Saute the onion until softened, about 3 minutes. Add the mushrooms and cook until they are browned and have released moisture, about 4-5 minutes. Add the cauliflower florets and cook until golden and crispy on the edges, approximately 8-10 minutes. Pour in the vegetable stock, top with mozzarella cheese (if desired) and cook for 2 more minutes to slightly reduce the sauce. Mix in thyme, one Tbsp. of parsley, garlic. Cook for another 30 seconds until fragrant. Season with salt and pepper, garnish with remaining parsley and serve hot.

CRISPY BROCCOLI CHEESE BITES

Ingredients:

- 2 cups fresh organic broccoli florets, finely chopped
- 1 cup shredded *Violife* organic cheddar cheese
- 1 cup gluten-free breadcrumbs
- 2 large eggs, beaten
- 1/2 cup grated *Violife* organic Parmesan cheese
- 1/4 cup finely chopped Shallot onion
- 1/4 cup King Arthur organic gluten-free flour
- 1 tsp. garlic powder
- 1/2 tsp. salt
- 1/4 tsp. black pepper

Directions:

Steam or blanch the broccoli florets until tender. Drain and chop finely. In a large bowl, combine the chopped broccoli, cheddar cheese, breadcrumbs, Parmesan cheese, onion, flour, garlic powder, salt, and black pepper. Pour in the beaten eggs and mix until the ingredients are well combined. Shape the mixture into small bite-sized balls or patties.

Preheat your oven to 375°F (190°C) and line a baking sheet with parchment paper. Arrange the bites on the prepared baking sheet and bake for 20-25 minutes or until golden brown and crispy. Allow the bites to cool slightly before serving.

GARLIC CHICKEN FRIED RICE

Ingredients:

- 1 Tbsp. olive oil
- 2 cups cooked brown rice, chilled
- 2 chicken breasts, diced
- 2 cloves garlic, minced
- 1 cup mixed vegetables (such as peas, carrots, green beans, broccoli)
- 2 eggs, beaten
- 2 Tbsps. tamari sauce
- 1 Tbsp. avocado oil
- Salt and pepper to taste
- Green onions for garnish (optional)

Directions:

In a large skillet or wok, heat olive oil over medium-high heat. Add diced chicken and minced garlic, and cook until chicken is cooked through and garlic is fragrant. Push the chicken to one side of the skillet and add beaten eggs to the other side. Scramble the eggs until fully cooked. Add mixed vegetables to the skillet and cook until they are tender. Add chilled rice to the skillet and stir-fry everything together, breaking up any clumps of rice. Pour tamari sauce and avocado oil over the rice mixture, and continue to stir-fry until everything is evenly coated. Season with salt and pepper to taste. Garnish with chopped green onions if desired. Serve hot and enjoy!

A flavorful twist on a classic dish! Tender chicken , fragrant garlic, and fluffy rice stir-fried to perfection.

GRILLED SALMON SKEWERS WITH CREAMY DILL YOGURT SAUCE

Ingredients:

For the Salmon Skewers:

- 1 1/2 pounds salmon fillets, cut into 1-inch cubes
- 2 Tbsps. olive oil
- 1 lemon, zest and juice
- 1 garlic clove, minced
- Salt and pepper to taste
- Wooden or metal skewers

For the Creamy Dill Yogurt Sauce:

- 1 cup dairy free Silk yogurt
- 2 Tbsps. chopped fresh dill
- 1 Tbsp. lemon juice
- 1 tsp. lemon zest
- 1 garlic clove, minced
- Salt and pepper to taste

Directions:

In a bowl, combine olive oil, lemon zest, lemon juice, minced garlic, salt, and pepper. Add the salmon cubes to the marinade and gently toss to coat. Let marinate for at least 30 minutes in the refrigerator. In a small bowl, mix together Greek yogurt, chopped dill, lemon juice, lemon zest, minced garlic, salt, and pepper until well combined.

Preheat the grill to medium-high heat. Thread the marinated salmon cubes onto skewers. Grill the skewers for 3-4 minutes on each side or until salmon is opaque and slightly charred. Serve the grilled salmon skewers with a generous drizzle or side of creamy dill yogurt sauce.

SPINACH RICOTTA STUFFED CHICKEN BREASTS

Ingredients:

- 4 boneless, skinless chicken breasts
- 1 cup *Kite Hill* ricotta cheese
- 1 cup fresh spinach, chopped
- 3 cloves garlic, minced
- 1/3 cup shallot onion, chopped
- 1/3 cup *Violife* Parmesan cheese, shredded
- Small handful of *Violife* mozzarella cheese
- Garlic powder, salt, and pepper to taste
- 1/2 cup cherry tomatoes
- 1/4 cup shredded *Violife* Parmesan cheese

Directions:

Cut chicken breasts down the middle on its side, but don't cut all the way through. Mix remaining ingredients except cherry tomatoes and 1/4 cup Parmesan cheese together. Stuff your mixture inside the chicken breasts and place in a glass baking dish. Bake at 425° for 35 minutes. When there are 10 minutes left, take out and top with sliced cherry tomatoes and Parmesan cheese. Bake the remaining 10 minutes.

You would add Prego Sensitive Recipe pasta sauce when you add the cherry tomatoes and Parmesan (optional).

ZUCCHINI PIZZA BITES

Ingredients:

- 2 large zucchinis, sliced into 1/2-inch rounds
- 1 cup marinara sauce (Organico Bello - Organic Gourmet Pasta Sauce or Organicville Pizza Sauce)
- 2 cups shredded *Violife* mozzarella cheese
- 1/2 cup mini pepperoni slices
- 1 Tbsp. Italian seasoning
- Olive oil for brushing
- Salt and pepper to taste
- Fresh basil leaves for garnish

Directions:

Preheat your oven to 400°F (200°C) and line a baking sheet with parchment paper. Brush both sides of the zucchini slices with olive oil and season with salt and pepper. Arrange the zucchini rounds on the prepared baking sheet. Spoon a small amount of marinara sauce on each zucchini round. Sprinkle shredded mozzarella cheese on top of the sauce. Add mini pepperoni slices to each zucchini round and sprinkle with Italian seasoning. Bake in the preheated oven for 10-12 minutes or until the cheese is melted and bubbly. Garnish with fresh basil leaves before serving.

MEDITERRANEAN CHICKEN ZUCCHINI BAKE

Ingredients:

- 3 boneless, skinless chicken breasts, cut into bite-sized pieces
- 2 medium zucchinis, sliced into rounds about 1/4 inch thick
- 1 pint cherry tomatoes, halved
- 1 red bell pepper, diced
- 1/2 Shallot onion, thinly sliced
- 3 garlic cloves, minced
- 1/4 cup olive oil or avocado oil
- 1 tsp. dried oregano
- 1 tsp. dried basil
- 1/2 tsp. dried thyme
- 1/2 cup crumbled *Violife* feta cheese
- Salt and pepper to taste
- Fresh parsley, chopped (optional)

Directions:

Preheat oven to 400°F (200°C). Grease a large baking dish with olive oil.

Combine the chicken pieces, zucchini slices, cherry tomatoes, red bell pepper, red onion, and minced garlic in a large bowl. Drizzle olive oil over the chicken and vegetables. Add oregano, basil, thyme, salt, and pepper. Toss until well coated. Transfer the mixture to the baking dish, spreading it out evenly. Bake for 25-30 minutes until chicken is cooked through and vegetables are tender. Sprinkle feta cheese over the top and bake for 5 more minutes until slightly melted. Garnish with chopped parsley if desired before serving.

A hearty and flavorful one-pan dish that combines juicy chicken, tender vegetables, and creamy feta cheese for a satisfying Mediterranean-inspired meal.

HONEY PINEAPPLE JALAPEÑO SALMON

Ingredients:

- 4 salmon fillets
- 1/2 cup pineapple chunks
- 2 Tbsps. jalapeños, sliced
- 1/4 cup raw local honey (if you have local supplier)
- 1/4 cup *San-J* gluten-free tamari soy sauce
- 2 Tbsps. lime juice
- 2 cloves garlic, minced
- 1 tsp. ginger, minced
- 2 Tbsps. olive oil
- Salt and pepper to taste
- Green onions, chopped (for garnish)

Directions:

In a bowl, whisk together honey, soy sauce, lime juice, minced garlic, and minced ginger. Place the salmon fillets in a shallow dish or a resealable plastic bag. Pour the marinade over the salmon, ensuring each fillet is well coated. Marinate in the refrigerator for at least 30 minutes.

In a large skillet, heat the olive oil over medium-high heat. Remove the salmon from the marinade and season with salt and pepper. Reserve the marinade. Place the salmon fillets in the skillet, skin side down. Cook for about 4-5 minutes per side, or until the salmon is cooked through and has a nice sear. Remove from the skillet and set aside.

In the same skillet, add the reserved marinade and bring it to a simmer. Cook for 2-3 minutes until the sauce thickens slightly. Stir in the pineapple chunks and sliced jalapeños. Cook for another 2 minutes until heated through.

Return the cooked salmon to the skillet, spooning the sauce over the fillets to coat them in the sticky, sweet, and spicy sauce. Garnish with chopped green onions. Serve hot with your favorite side dish.

A sweet and spicy salmon dish that's bursting with tropical flavors!

CREAMY SPINACH TOMATO SPAGHETTI

Ingredients:

- 1/2 cup *Violife* sour cream
- 2 cloves garlic, minced
- 2 Tbsps. butter - Country Crock Dairy Free Vegan Plant Butter with Olive Oil
- Fresh spinach leaves (about 4 cups)
- 8 oz. (1 pkg.) of *Jovial* spaghetti noodles
- 1/2 cup oil-packed sun-dried tomatoes, drained and chopped (reserve some oil)
- 1 small red onion, finely chopped
- 1/2 tsp. crushed red pepper flakes
- Salt and pepper to taste
- 1 cup low-sodium vegetable or chicken broth
- 1/2 cup grated *Violife* Parmesan cheese

Directions:

Place spinach leaves in a large colander. Boil salted water, cook pasta according to the package instructions. Drain the pasta over the spinach to wilt it. Heat reserved sun-dried tomato oil in a skillet. Sauté the onion and sun-dried tomatoes, then add garlic, red pepper flakes, salt, and pepper. Add broth and reduce by half. Stir in sour cream, Parmesan cheese, and butter until creamy. Combine the spaghetti and wilted spinach with the sauce in the skillet and toss until coated. Garnish with extra Parmesan if desired.

This works great for big family gatherings.

CHICKEN MUSHROOM AND SPINACH LASAGNA

Ingredients:

- 2 1/2 Tbsps. olive oil
- 1 cup chopped Shallot onion
- 2 Tbsps. minced garlic
- 8 oz. white mushrooms, thinly sliced
- 1 tsp. dried basil
- 1 tsp. dried oregano
- 1/2 tsp. red pepper flakes
- 1 1/4 tsps. kosher salt, divided
- 1 (6 oz.) bag fresh baby spinach
- 2 cups shredded cooked chicken
- 2 cups low-sodium chicken stock
- 1/4 cup *King Arthur* gluten-free flour
- 2 cups almond milk
- 1/4 tsp. nutmeg
- 1/2 cup shredded *Violife* Parmesan cheese
- 8 no-boil *Barilla* Gluten-Free Oven-Ready lasagna noodles
- 1 1/4 cups shredded *Violife* mozzarella cheese

Directions:

Preheat the oven to 375°F (190°C). Heat a large sauté pan over medium-high heat. Add olive oil, then the onions, garlic, mushrooms, basil, oregano, red pepper flakes, and 1/4 tsp. of salt. Sauté for 5 minutes or until the mushrooms soften, stirring occasionally. Stir in the spinach and cook until wilted and all its moisture has evaporated. Remove the pan from the heat and stir in the cooked chicken. Set aside.

In a small bowl, make a slurry by whisking together 1/2 cup chicken stock with flour until it reaches a thick, milky consistency. Set aside.

In a small saucepan, combine the remaining 1 1/2 cups chicken stock, milk, nutmeg, and 1 tsp. of salt. Bring to a slow simmer over medium heat, stirring occasionally. Once the mixture starts to bubble around the edges, add the slurry while whisking continuously. Simmer until thickened, about 5-8 minutes, whisking occasionally. Stir in Parmesan cheese and remove from heat.

Pour 1/2 cup of the sauce into the bottom of a 10×10 inch square baking dish. Top with 2 lasagna noodles, 1 cup of the chicken mixture, 1 cup of sauce, and 1/4 cup of mozzarella, ensuring the noodles are covered with sauce. Press them down lightly if needed. Repeat the layers three more times with noodles, chicken, sauce, and cheese. The last layer should have slightly more sauce and the remaining cheese on top. Cover the baking dish with aluminum foil and bake for 25 minutes. Uncover and bake for an additional 15 minutes. If desired, broil for 2-3 minutes to achieve a golden brown top. Let the lasagna stand for 15-20 minutes before cutting and serving.

A savory and creamy lasagna packed with tender chicken, mushrooms, and spinach, layered with rich cheese and a delicious white sauce. Perfect for a comforting dinner that everyone will love!

MUSHROOM RAVIOLI WITH SPINACH

Ingredients:

- 1 cup mushrooms, white or bella, chopped
- 2 cups fresh spinach
- 1/2 cup heavy cream (*Silk* Dairy Free Heavy Whipping Cream)
- 1/4 cup *Violife* Parmesan cheese, grated
- 1/2 cup chicken broth
- 1 Tbsp. olive oil
- 1/2 tsp. salt
- 1/4 tsp. black pepper
- 1 pkg. (9 oz.) *La Pasta* Gluten-Free Mushroom Ravioli

Directions:

Boil ravioli according to package instructions. Drain and set aside. Heat olive oil in a large skillet over medium heat. Add mushrooms, salt, and pepper. Cook until mushrooms are soft. Stir in spinach and cook until wilted. Pour in chicken broth and heavy cream. Stir and bring to a simmer. Add cooked ravioli to the skillet. Toss gently to coat in sauce. Sprinkle Parmesan cheese over the top. Serve warm.

MARINADE RECIPES FOR CHICKEN

Directions:

All marinades recommended for 1-1.5 lbs. boneless chicken thighs (or turkey breast). Place meat breasts or thighs in a Ziplock bag, large bowl, or container. In a small bowl or jar, mix together the marinade ingredients. Pour over the meat and allow to sit for at least 30 minutes before baking, pan cooking or air frying, or package in a Ziplock bag and store in the freezer for later use.

Chipotle Chicken Marinade Ingredients:

- 2 Tbsps. olive oil
- 2 tsps. adobo sauce (from a can of chipotle peppers)
- 1/2 tsp. paprika
- 2 tsps. brown sugar
- 2 cloves garlic, minced
- 1/4 tsp. salt

Honey Mustard Chicken Marinade Ingredients:

- 3 Tbsps. Dijon mustard
- 2 Tbsps. honey
- 2 clove garlic, minced, or 1/2 tsp. garlic granules
- 1 tsp. onion powder
- 1/2 tsp. each sea salt and pepper

Greek Chicken Marinade Ingredients:

- 3 Tbsps. olive oil
- 3 Tbsps. lemon juice
- 3 garlic cloves, minced
- 1 1/2 Tbsps. dried oregano
- 1 Tbsp. red wine vinegar
- 1/2 tsp. salt
- 1/2 tsp. black pepper

Fajita Chicken Marinade Ingredients:

- 3 Tbsps. olive oil
- Juice of one lime
- 1 1/2 tsps. chili powder
- 1 tsp. garlic powder
- 1/2 tsp. smoked paprika
- 1/2 tsp. onion powder
- 1/2 tsp. cumin
- 1/2 tsp. dried oregano
- 1/2 tsp. each salt and black pepper

Teriyaki Chicken Marinade Ingredients:

- 1/4 cup soy sauce
- 2 tsps. fresh grated ginger
- 1/2 tsp. sriracha
- 2 cloves garlic minced
- 3 Tbsps. maple syrup
- 2 Tbsps. chopped green onion
- 2 Tbsps. rice vinegar

DESSERTS & SNACKS

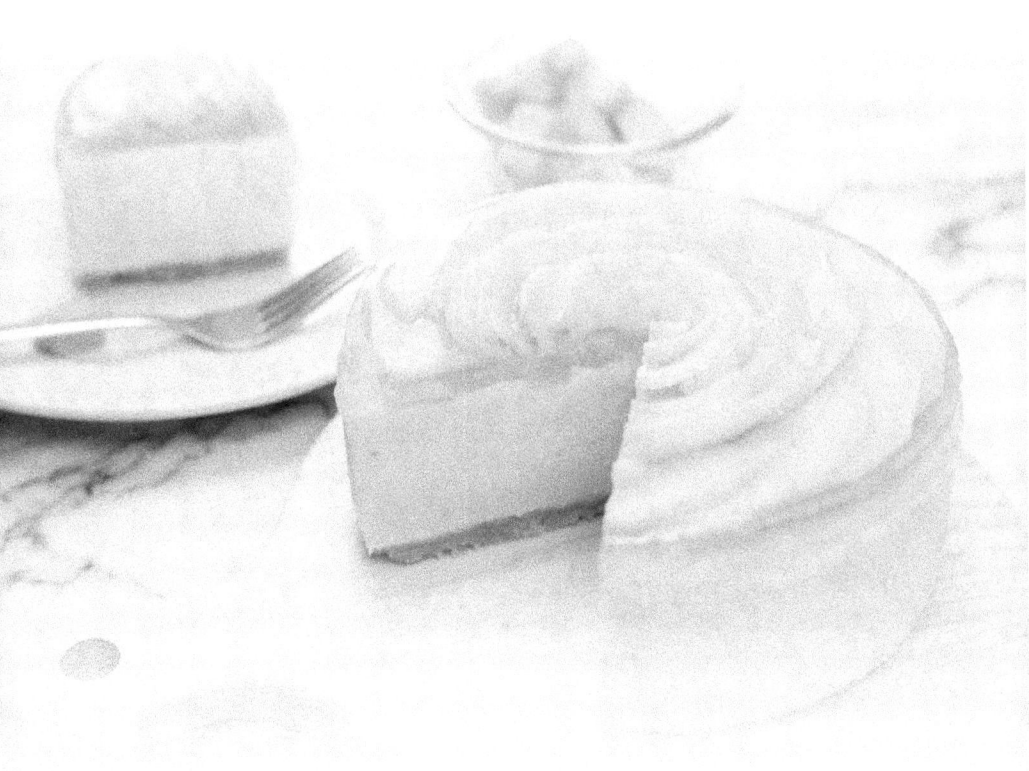

FRUIT PROTEIN BALLS

Ingredients:

- 1 1/2 cups oats (gluten free)
- 1/2 pkg. dried blueberries (or any dried fruit)
- 1 cup gluten-free peanut butter
- 1/4 cup crushed white chocolate chips
- 40g vanilla protein power (1 scoop)
- 1/4 cup raw honey
- 1/4 maple syrup

Directions:

Mix well and make into small balls.

YOUR MANGO CHEESECAKE DELIGHT

Ingredients:

- 1 1/2 cups graham cracker crumbs
- 1/4 cup unsalted *Violife* butter, melted
- 3 cups *Violife* cream cheese, at room temperature
- 1 cup granulated sugar
- 1 cup mango puree
- 3 large eggs
- 1 teaspoon vanilla extract
- 1/2 cup *Violife* sour cream
- Fresh mango slices for garnish
- Edible flowers for garnish (optional)

Directions:

Preheat oven to 325°. Combine graham cracker crumbs with melted butter and press into the bottom of a spring-form pan to form the crust. In a large mixing bowl, beat the cream cheese until smooth. Add sugar and mango puree, and continue to beat until well combined. Add eggs one at a time, beating well after each addition. Stir in vanilla extract. Fold in sour cream until the mixture is smooth. Pour the cream cheese mixture over the crust in the spring-form pan. Bake for 55 minutes, or until the center is just set. Allow to cool to room temperature, then refrigerate for at least 4 hours or overnight. Garnish with fresh mango slices and edible flowers before serving.

CHERRY CHEESECAKE FLUFF

Ingredients:

For the Fluff:
- 1 (8 oz) pkg. *Violife* cream cheese, softened
- 1 cup powdered sugar
- 1 teaspoon vanilla extract
- 2 cups whipped topping (like *Truwhip Vegan* or *Coco Whip*), thawed
- 1 (21 oz) can cherry pie filling

For the Crumble:
- 1 cup graham cracker crumbs (*Schär*, *Pamela's*, and *Kinnikinnick* brands are gluten-free)
- 1/4 cup unsalted *Violife* butter, melted
- 2 tablespoons sugar

Directions:

Mix graham cracker crumbs, melted butter, and sugar in a bowl until well combined. Set aside.

In a large mixing bowl, beat the cream cheese until smooth. Add powdered sugar and vanilla extract, continuing to beat until well blended. Fold in the whipped topping gently until the mixture is smooth.

To assemble the layers in your serving dish, layer half of the crumble mixture at the bottom. Spread the cream cheese mixture over the crumble layer evenly. Top with the cherry pie filling, spreading it out to cover the cream cheese layer completely. Finish by sprinkling the remaining crumble mixture over the cherry layer. Refrigerate for at least 2 hours before serving to allow the flavors to meld and the dessert to firm up.

FRUIT BLISS CHEESECAKE

Ingredients:

For the Crust:
- 1 1/2 cups crushed digestive biscuits
- 1/3 cup unsalted *Violife* butter, melted
- 2 tablespoons granulated sugar

For the Cheesecake Mixture:
- 4 cups *Violife* cream cheese, softened
- 1 cup granulated sugar
- 2 teaspoons pure vanilla extract
- 4 large eggs
- 1 cup *Violife* sour cream

For the Fruit Layer:
- 1 cup fresh peaches, thinly sliced
- 1 cup fresh raspberries

Directions:

Preheat your oven to 325°. Mix the biscuit crumbs with melted butter and sugar, then press firmly into the bottom of a greased 9-inch spring-form pan.

In a bowl, blend cream cheese with sugar and vanilla until smooth. Incorporate eggs one at a time, then fold in the sour cream.

Pour half of the cheesecake mixture over the crust. Layer with sliced peaches and raspberries, then top with the remaining mixture. Arrange additional peach slices and raspberries on top. Bake for 50 minutes, or until set. Let cool, then chill for at least 4 hours in the refrigerator. Garnish with whipped cream, fresh peach slices, raspberries, and mint before serving.

BROWNIE BOMBS

Ingredients:

- 3/4 cup *Violife* butter, softened
- 3/4 cup brown sugar
- 1/4 cup white sugar
- 2 tablespoons almond milk
- 1 teaspoon vanilla extract
- 2 cups almond flour
- Pinch of salt
- 2 cups miniature chocolate chips, divided
- 1 pkg. gluten-free brownie mix, baked and cooled
- 1 pkg. chocolate almond bark

Directions:

In a stand mixer, beat together softened butter, brown sugar, and white sugar until smooth. Mix in milk and vanilla extract until well blended. Gradually add all-purpose flour and salt to the mixture, mixing until a soft dough forms. Stir in 1 cup of miniature chocolate chips until evenly distributed.

On a foil-lined baking sheet, shape scant tablespoon-sized balls of cookie dough. Freeze the dough balls for 1 hour.

Cook the brownies according to package instructions, then cut the cooled brownies into 1-inch squares. Flatten each square and place a frozen dough ball in the center. Wrap the brownie around the dough, forming a ball. Freeze the wrapped balls for an additional 30 minutes.

Melt the chocolate almond bark according to package instructions. Dip each brownie bomb into the melted chocolate, allowing any excess to drip off. Place the dipped bombs on foil and sprinkle with the remaining miniature chocolate chips. Chill the Chocolate Chip Cookie Dough Brownie Bombs until the chocolate coating is set. Store the bombs in an airtight container in the fridge or freezer until ready to enjoy.

CARAMEL CHEESECAKE BARS

Ingredients:

- 2 cups graham cracker crumbs
- 1/4 cup sugar
- 1/2 cup *Violife* butter, melted
- 8 ounces *Violife* cream cheese
- 1 1/2 cups sugar
- 2 teaspoons vanilla extract
- 4 eggs
- 1/2 cup *Violife* sour cream
- 1/2 cup brown sugar
- 6 tablespoons *Violife* butter
- 14 ounces sweetened condensed *Andre Prost* coconut milk
- 2 tablespoons corn syrup
- 1 teaspoon vanilla extract

Directions:

Preheat oven to 350°.

For the crust, combine graham cracker crumbs, sugar, and melted butter. Press into the bottom of a 9×13 inch baking dish sprayed with nonstick cooking spray. Set aside.

For the filling, beat together cream cheese, sugar, and vanilla until smooth. Beat in eggs, one at a time. Add sour cream and mix until smooth. Pour over prepared crust, smooth top and bake for 50 minutes. Turn off the oven, open the door and let the cheesecake sit in the warm oven for 15 minutes. Remove and let cool for an hour.

For the caramel topping, combine brown sugar and butter in a saucepan over medium heat. Stir until the butter is melted and sugar is dissolved. Whisk in condensed milk, corn syrup, and vanilla and bring to a boil, stirring continuously. Boil until the caramel reaches 225°. Let caramel cool in the pan for 3-5 minutes, then pour over cheesecake. Smooth and let set until cool. Cut into squares and serve.

You can store these Caramel Cheesecake Bars in an airtight container in the refrigerator for up to 3-4 days.

WHITE CHOCOLATE STRAWBERRY CHEESECAKE BITES

Ingredients:

- 1 cup crushed graham crackers
- 3 tablespoons unsalted butter (dairy/gluten-free), melted
- 1 pkg. (8 oz) *Violife* cream cheese, softened
- 1/4 cup granulated sugar
- 1/2 teaspoon vanilla extract
- 1/2 cup white chocolate chips, melted
- 1/2 cup fresh strawberries, finely chopped
- Extra strawberries and white chocolate chips, for garnish

Directions:

In a mixing bowl, combine crushed graham crackers and melted butter until the mixture resembles wet sand. Press the graham cracker mixture into the bottom of a silicone mini muffin pan to form the bases.

In another bowl, beat the cream cheese, sugar, and vanilla extract until smooth. Fold the melted white chocolate into the cream cheese mixture until well combined. Stir in the finely chopped strawberries. Spoon the cream cheese mixture over the graham cracker bases, filling each to the top. Refrigerate for at least 2 hours, or until set. Once set, gently remove the cheesecake bites from the silicone pan. Garnish each bite with a small piece of strawberry and a drizzle of melted white chocolate before serving.

www.ingramcontent.com/pod-product-compliance
Lightning Source LLC
Chambersburg PA
CBHW072210070526
44585CB00015B/1279